A New Name

ivp

A New Name

Grace and healing for anorexia

Emma Scrivener

INTER-VARSITY PRESS
Norton Street, Nottingham NG7 3HR, England
Email: ivp@ivpbooks.com
Website: www.ivpbooks.com

© Emma Scrivener, 2012

First published 2012
Reprinted 2013

British Library Cataloguing in Publication Data
A catalogue record for this book is available from the British Library.

ISBN: 978–1–84474–586–9

Set in Chapperal 12/15pt
Typeset in Great Britain by CRB Associates, Potterhanworth, Lincolnshire
Printed and bound in Great Britain by MPG Books Ltd, Bodmin, Cornwall

*Inter-Varsity Press publishes Christian books that are true to the Bible and that
communicate the gospel, develop discipleship and strengthen the church for its
mission in the world.*

*Inter-Varsity Press is closely linked with the Universities and Colleges Christian
Fellowship, a student movement connecting Christian Unions in universities and
colleges throughout Great Britain, and a member movement of the International
Fellowship of Evangelical Students. Website: www.uccf.org.uk*

For Glen,
who showed me Jesus
and never gave up

Contents

Acknowledgments

So many people have advised and prayed for me with this book, but I'd like to say a special thanks to Eleanor for championing it, Judy and Bethan for their wisdom and encouragement, Glen (for everything) and Rachel – just for being her.

Introduction

In my hand I held a sliver of bread. I turned it over in my palms, smelled it, stroked it. I imagined how it tasted. The feel of it in my mouth, my stomach. I traced it with my yellowed fingers. The hands of a skeleton, tipped with blackened nails I hadn't painted.

My head throbbed and, though it was the middle of summer, I was shivering with cold. I always felt cold, right to the bone. I lifted my T-shirt. Traced the skeleton, so close to the skin. Not there yet, but it was coming. Just a little more effort. Shave a little more off.

Unless, of course, I'd gained weight in the last half-hour. Best to check, just in case. I pulled myself up, waiting for the dizziness to pass. Squashed the bread and smelt my palms. I was ravenous. My head swam, but my stomach, hollowed and hardened, was silent. I'd rather die than eat.

Think of something else. Anything. That's it – breathe. Now, take a step. You can do it. Stop being so lazy. Count to ten – one, two, three . . .

Moving forward, a stab of pain cut across my chest. Not again! This time, however, it didn't pass. I felt like I was suffocating and tried to gulp down lungfuls of air. My legs crumpled and I fell, hard upon the floor. Something was bleeding, but the cool tiles felt clean against my face. I wanted to get up, but I was tired, so tired. How pleasant it would be to stay here, forever. But the scales, just across the hall, were beckoning.

Sucking in my cheeks, I tried to pull myself upright. My brain barked orders, but the limbs remained still, twisted and splayed like a rag doll tossed to one side. It was a curious sensation, like seeing myself from a great height. But I couldn't stay here, flesh spilling across the floor. It had been over an hour since my last run. I had to go to the bathroom. I had to weigh myself.

Using my feet as a lever, I coughed and took another breath. Then I pushed away from the wall. Palms outstretched, I dragged my torso across the stone. Bit by bit, I inched forward. Fat. Lazy. Cow. A sharp intake of breath as my ribs jarred on the cracks. I paused, then blinked. Outside I could hear traffic and the sound of voices, but they seemed very far away. I brushed a clump of hair from my eyes, watching with mild interest as it came off in my hands. It was still cold, but I'd wet myself and the dampness in my legs felt soothing and warm.

I was twenty-eight years old. A talented student at Bible college. I led a thriving Sunday school. I'd been married for four years to a church minister in training. And I was slowly but surely killing myself.

I blacked out.

* * *

In the face of an eating disorder, one question stands out: *Why?* Why me? Why *my* daughter, why *my* wife . . . *my* brother, *my* friend?

As we tell our stories, we naturally seek a villain, someone or something to blame. A school bully, a body-obsessed media, bad parenting or some childhood trauma. These may well be contributors, but if drawn on a pie chart, they would make up only part of the whole. Instead, many factors come into play: culture, environment, physiology, family, personality type, life experiences, even geography. Some can be predicted and managed. Others cannot. Some are a result of the choices that we have made. Others are decisions that have been made for us – whatever their motivation.

As I survey the wreckage from two decades fighting anorexia, I feel like I'm performing the wrong script. This is not where I planned to be. It's not the romantic comedy I'd rehearsed for as a child – and where's Brad Pitt? Instead, I'm trapped in a Russian submarine tragedy and I can't even read the subtitles.

On the other hand, there's a nagging sense that I've stage-managed my own demise. Perhaps the blame is entirely mine. I followed my own directions, even when others begged me to stop. Now the lights have dimmed and I'm left alone in the darkness.

So which is it? Am I a willing perpetrator or a helpless victim? Is this sickness – or is it sin?

As I write my story, I'm pulled in two directions. I want to defend myself and to tear myself down. Sometimes I'll do both. You may be tempted to do the same, and of course you must draw your own conclusions. But I suspect that the truth – as close as I can tell it – lies somewhere else.

Jesus Christ calls himself a Doctor for sick sinners. And I am both. I'm sick – helpless in the face of a condition that overpowers me. I'm *also* a sinner – deliberately choosing my way over his. Despite this, he loves me just the same. So this is not just 'my' story. It's the story of his work in my life.

1 Rare

I was born Emma Sloan. I've always considered it a 'good' name. Simple, easy to spell and with no complicated add-ons. 'Emma Sloan' could be a foxy secret agent. Or a brilliant physicist and part-time model. Wishful thinking, of course.

But after all, what's in a name?

In one sense, nothing. I'm more than just a label, right? Yet, in another, I'm not so sure. The question of name has defined my life so far; in this, I suspect, I'm not alone. All of us want to know who we are and where we fit. It's an enquiry that underpins everything we do, from the moment we wake, till our head hits the pillow. It's the motivation behind our choices – from what we wear to where we go and how we relate to other people. If I sat down beside you and asked who you are, what would you say?

A wife?

A father? A daughter?

An accountant?

A frustrated pop star? A cat-lover?

. . . Or something else?

It's not an easy question – in part, because there are so many 'right' answers. From cradle to grave, we are bombarded by names. The names that we choose. Our married names. Avatars and stage names. Online identities. Pen names.

Then there are the names that are chosen for us. Family names. Echoes from the schoolyard. Or nicknames, bestowed with affection by friends or lovers. There are names we'd like to forget. Hurtful names, tossed like mud in the playground or the office. Names that stick and won't wash off.

Wherever we go, competing voices are clamouring to tell us who we are. The question is this: Which ones do we believe? Whom can we trust? And what happens when the answers and the reality don't match up?

I'm convinced that we've all been given a true name, one that tells us who and what we are. It's not the name we build for ourselves, nor is it conferred by others. It's a name that's given to us by the Lord. When we accept it – when we accept him – the hiding, the searching and the striving can finally stop. We can rest. In him we can find our true purpose, meaning and identity.

Childhood

I was raised in Belfast, the eldest of three siblings. My brother Michael says that he got the looks, my sister Ruth the brains and me the morals. I like to think he's joking, but I'll let you draw your own conclusions.

Whatever you think of 'birth-order' psychology, I've definitely got certain traits. I'm conscientious, bossy and driven. Recently, I completed the '*Star Wars* personality test' – a scientifically proven indicator of character. My profile matched that of 'the Emperor', while my husband was identified as 'Princess Leia'. This upset us both. In case you don't know the film, the Emperor is the bossiest and meanest character in the galaxy. In his defence, he gets things done . . . but he is a little controlling. I blame the parents – of whom, more later.

If we could rewind to ten-year-old Emma, whom would we see?

A good girl. Slim, pale, fidgety. Thoughtful. Restless, energetic, lots of hair, knobbly knees. Far from a super-model in waiting, but passable enough.

Dad says that I was always a 'joiner'. Whatever was happening, I had to take part. It's terminally uncool, but I couldn't help myself. I would talk to everyone (including trees) and happily trotted off with complete strangers. Other people fascinated me – their experiences, their mannerisms, the way they thought and the things they said. On their own they were like human puzzles, waiting to be unlocked. Groups, however, were different: overwhelming, even frightening. Confronted by these sprawling continents of humanity, I would siphon off individuals, then colonize them one by one. This pattern continued throughout school, where I'd have just one best friend (as well as a whole cast of imaginary ones). Even today, I'd rather get to know one person or topic deeply, than spread myself thinly. Small talk still seems like a waste of time, a distraction from what is really important.

This intensity characterizes almost everything I do: from friendships to conversation, work to rest. In my world, 'hobbies' quickly become obsessions. It's how I've always been – all or nothing, double-concentrate, personality and need spilling out onto paper and people.

As a child, I saw life as an adventure – magical and addictive. Even the shopping centres seemed beautiful – brimming with bright colours, sounds and scents that left me winded but hungry for more. I was filled with inarticulate and insatiable longings. Nothing – whether time or money or food or friendship – was ever enough. I remember standing in the garden, cradling an apple core, and wondering as it decayed in my hands. In my palms I held the key to the universe, but I couldn't unlock it. What did it mean? I wanted to hold it, to capture its essence, its secret. But it always remained just out of reach.

Everything in my upbringing and culture resists it – but from the earliest age I felt . . . extraordinary. I know how this sounds: ridiculous and overblown. But I had an overwhelming sense of the importance of life and my place in it. Little things – the shape of a leaf or the taste of a strawberry – could move me to tears. I believed that I was special, set apart for a purpose I could neither express nor understand. Invincible too. In my head I scaled mountains, watched planets collide, felt the grass growing, the swell of the ocean under my feet. At night my brain refused to shut down, whirring instead over the minutiae and mystery of existence.

Mostly my body was an uncomplicated extension of myself. But, sometimes, I felt a disjunction between the thoughts that raced ahead and the limbs that lagged behind. I remember reading about dragons and concluding that flight was simply a case of mind over matter. Armed with limitless self-belief, I leapt repeatedly from the garden fence, expecting to soar like an eagle over the houses. Inevitably, I would plummet to the pavement, bruised and bewildered, but determined to get it right next time round.

They said at school, 'She reads too much' – and perhaps they were right. I've always loved words. The shape of them – their curls and spirals. The way they sound, their see-saw, echoing cadences. With language, unlike life, there's no right or wrong, black and white. Instead it's a glorious multiplicity of meaning – to paraphrase MacNeice, a 'drunken savour-ing of things being various'.[1] I'm a product of my place, too. Irish literature courses like blood through my veins, filling them with warfare and poetry, magic and questions. Searching for answers, I would plunder the local library, saturating my senses with pirates and Vikings, wizards and castles. My head was permanently bowed – even at school, where, ever the rebel, I was reprimanded for reading under the table. Determined to finish the chapter, I waged bitter but futile warfare against sleep. But my mind was inevitably defeated by a body that couldn't keep up.

I swallowed books like a drowning man and, in turn, my words spilled out. I was fired with stories, dreams and poetry, but my fingers cramped before they could be captured on paper. In primary school the teachers said I had a 'gift' for writing. Test sheets showed my English abilities were off the charts. (My maths skills were also off the scale, though unfortunately in the opposite direction.)

This was a double-edged sword. In some ways it's good to feel different: exciting and liberating too. You see the world through a slightly different lens. Feelings come in technicolour – grief and pity and anger and love. When you're happy, you're unbeatable and nothing is beyond your reach. But that's not the full story. Sometimes it's just tiring and lonely. More than anything, you want to be accepted and to belong. To feel it's OK just to be you.

Sponge-like, my heart soaked up praise – but it was never enough. The warm glow of achievement faded before the exam grades had dried. Approval was addictive, but ultimately unsatisfying. Each time I had to do better, to score higher. I competed against myself – but I was never good enough.

Even at primary school, I worked through the night, writing and rewriting stories, essays and journals. It wasn't my parents or my teachers pushing me on. Those drives and hungers came from me – and they've always been there. I didn't know what they were called or where to put them. What I did know was this: they were too much. *I* was too much – too inward, too intense. I felt awkward, even shameful. I needed to be contained.

For this reason, writing was important. It was a reservoir into which I poured my excess – something that marked me out – but in a positive way. Speech could be slippery, but writing was a sanctuary, of silence and space. When I wrote, I connected with others and felt myself heard. It was as necessary and as natural as breathing.

In the face of my anxieties, I longed to fit in but also to stand out. It's a perverse sort of selfishness – pride allied to self-doubt. I wanted to be the best and to shine the brightest. Why? Because I knew that I wasn't. In everything, I fell short of the mark. When I wrote, I laid myself bare: I was exposed to both criticism and praise. When I handed in my papers, it wasn't just the assignments that were being graded. It was *me*. This was why it mattered.

Welcome to the family

It's within our families that we first learn who we are. I've spent years laughing at my parents, but I now realize that I've become them. We Sloans are a formidable unit – a long and distinguished line of talkers, all itching to say their piece. So let me introduce them to you, starting with my parents – Stanton and Linda.

It's hard to imagine my parents were ever young, even though photos attest to an attractive (albeit fashion-challenged) couple. Mum had three brothers and was the baby of the family. Her father, Robert Black, trained as a French polisher and was a gentle man of stillness and strength. In contrast, Granny or 'Mina' overflowed with words and laughter. She cannily signed all the grandkids' cards with the words 'you're my favourite' – but we believed her nonetheless. Their house, a warm fug of comfort and activity, was a little two-up, two-down terrace in east Belfast: small but carefully kept.

Dad tells me his childhood was at a time before contraception and, as the eldest boy in a family of seven, I can well believe it. He lived on the other side of town, in west Belfast. Bertha Sloan, his mum, smoked like a chimney and could talk for Ireland. His dad, Joshua, worked as a fitter and looked like Charlton Heston. A colossus of testosterone, he was loved and feared in equal measure, and his temper was the stuff of legend. Their cat discovered this to her cost when she left a smelly deposit in his slippers. Picking her up by the tail, Granda Sloan narrowed his eyes and drop-kicked her into next door's garden. The poor feline survived, but learned quickly from her mistake.

Mum and Dad first met and dated, briefly, when they were sixteen. The relationship didn't last. During this time, civil conflict was at its height, and they lived at opposite ends of town, so meeting was difficult. In the interim, both left school, Mum to work as an accountant, Dad as a researcher. They met again several years later, at a New Year's Eve party. By this time, Mum was dating someone else. 'Poor George' (as he's now fondly known) was one of Belfast's great romantics. He even bought her a frying pan, as a pledge of his undying love. This was impressive, but no match for Stanton. Dad spotted her at the party, marched up and delivered the now-famous line: 'Leave him and come with me.' She did – and, aged twenty-one, they were married. In March 1978 I was born, followed two years later by my sister, Ruth, and finally Michael, in 1982. Everyone was happy – especially Granny, who kept the frying pan.

My family have always been close. At times I found it hard to say where I ended and they began. As I grew up, my parents were my best friends, an extension of myself. On our wedding day, Dad eyeballed my new hubby and reminded him that, while he was welcomed into the family, I was and always would be a 'Sloan'. It was a joke, I think. Yet the point still stands: names and families matter.

Families are complicated. They shape and brand us with inescapable markers of identity, from comic timing to knobbly knees (a double curse from my mother). In them we play games of deadly seriousness, we form alliances and hierarchies, we assign and take on roles: the black sheep, the scapegoat, the golden child. We fight together and we love together too. We are knitted together, but we tear one another apart. For this reason, each family needs boundaries, to keep those inside safe, and the 'bad guys' out.

Every group, from the smallest tribe to the sprawling superpower, operates according to certain codes. Ours was no different. The Protestant work ethic ran through us like a stick of rock – a talisman against profligacy, gambling and drunkenness. My parents were the first in their families to attend university. They were bright, but worked hard to give us a quality of life that they had never enjoyed. They also taught us the importance of certain rules. We learned, for example, the value of obedience and respect for authority. It was OK to make mistakes, but never to lie. 'Sloans,' my dad would say, 'always tell the truth.' When we were caught, he would sometimes line us up in the hall, until one of us owned up. This was a brilliant system, largely because my sister, unable to bear the tension, would inevitably confess – regardless of her innocence.

Another lesson my parents taught me was that men and women, though equal, are different. Despite the vagaries of culture and fashion, in our house at least, gender was not interchangeable. In their generation, the man's job was to protect and provide for wife and family, while she in turn looked after him and built the home. Thus, when we were born, Mum stayed at home to take care of us, while Dad went out to work. Later, however, Mum retrained, becoming a teacher and then a headmistress. It was a great achievement, but impossible without Dad's encouragement and support.

Anchors

Especially as a child, my sense of my father was of his strength. He ruled our house and therefore the world.

At home we were untouchable, loved and safe. Nothing could shake him. Nothing could pluck me from the shelter of his arms. Guardians of knowledge, he and Mum were my best friends, my mentors and my world. To them I pledged unwavering allegiance, and in turn I knew myself to be unassailably loved and secure. My faith in them was unshakeable and absolute. In the same way, my father looked up to his dad and my mum's father.

Faced with an uncertain world, our parents ground us and act as our anchors. This means that when we lose them, we also lose a piece of ourselves. One of my most vivid memories is of when Granda Black died. He and Granny were united by a quiet but fierce love and, in fifty years of marriage, they hadn't spent a single night apart. Granny's friends were taking a trip to Scotland and talked her into going, just for a few days. While she was gone, Granda was taken into hospital for a routine operation. He never woke up.

On that day, I remember stumbling, white-faced, into the kitchen. Dad was there, silently doubled over the sink, shoulders heaving in grief. It was the first time I had seen him cry. My daddy, the foundation of the world, last bastion of strength and safety, had broken. With all my heart, I wanted to make him better, but there was a terrible loneliness to his grief. I backed, unspeaking, from the room.

It seemed that there was something bigger than my dad, something terrible that neither he nor I could control. Death had entered our world and, with it, the old certainties were swept away.

Words and people

In his strength and his silence, my dad typifies the Northern Irish man. But, as a people, we can be somewhat schizophrenic – caught between opposing and sometimes competing desires. Reticence is part of our national character, but contrasts with a natural gregariousness, a passion for words and relationships.

We are renowned for being both tight-fisted and open-handed. Perhaps it's because we've had to fight for what we've got. My generation have reaped the benefits of political and economic prosperity, but both peace and plenty are comparatively recent developments. Mum and Dad are a good example. In comparison to my grandparents, they have plenty of money and both are generous to a fault. Nonetheless, Dad still thinks that a haircut costs £1.50, and Mum will travel across town to secure a three-for-one offer on orange juice.

The Irish have a strength and a dark humour that's born out of struggle – whether against famine or war. Yet it comes at a cost: as history testifies, we rarely forgive or forget. Time mutes the stench and stain of blood, but the old scars remain. This siege mentality, combined with our island status, lends us a certain defensiveness. We know who and what we are. We're Northern Irish, and it's 'us' against the world. The past – a bold and bloody tapestry of intertwined stories, rivalries and relationships – won't stay silent. It won't let us go.

Perhaps this helps to explain our dislike of difference – a shared suspicion of the one who draws attention to himself, who's 'all mouth and no trousers'. We have a long tradition of telling stories against ourselves, and dishing out what's known as a 'joke with a jag' – a steely criticism candied in jest.

The Irish are known as a nation of 'blarney': silver-tongued charmers with the 'gift of the gab'. But don't be fooled. Our words can act as defences as much as invitations. While we raise up the balladeers, we can gun down the big-talkers.

As all writers know, language can build barricades as well as bridges. We may flood you with words, but they are often barriers against emotion and weakness:

'Don't be so ridiculous.'
'Pull your head in.'
'Wise up – it was only a joke.'

We create diversions and games of distraction:

'Sure, never worry.'
'Ach, it'll be fine – don't dwell on it.'
'No sense getting het up.'

Such phrases serve as warnings as well as reassurance. Don't lift the lid. Don't make a fuss. A kind of verbal ping-pong, where concerns are batted away before they can be voiced. An unspoken warning: keep it together – whatever's simmering beneath the surface.

Place

In a small community, appearances are important. I think of my granny, sluicing the steps of her tiny terraced house every morning without fail. Those steps were the frontispiece of her world and ours, indicators of physical and even moral cleanliness.

When everything is whispered but nothing is secret, what you're seen to do can matter as much as the reality. Judgments and opinion weigh heavily, even if nothing is said. We can suppress them, ignore them, and even drown them in a pint (or seven) of the black stuff. But what's repressed inevitably resurfaces, whether as banter or bullets.

Religion and politics were topics that we didn't discuss at home – but they were unavoidable nonetheless. On the streets and in the schools, terrorists detonated their volleyed fury – with both sides claiming divine sanction. If you were Protestant, then you were probably Unionist. If you were Catholic, you were probably Republican. In both garrisons, the living and the dead jostled to be heard. History was in the present – graffitied indelibly across walls and lives. This meant there were places – physical and psychological – where you just couldn't go. Instead, we were like jealous cats, staking out our territory.

Geography matters, especially in Ireland. Our contested soil reflects boundaries that both imprison and protect. Checkpoints, barricades and borders demarcated the urban landscape – yet beyond the city lay the craggy splendour of the coast, sprawling and untamed. It's a striking contrast. On one hand stood the grey streets and skies, the bricks and bombs, the rows of shuttered tenement houses. Then there were the whistling dunes, the valleys and fields: amber and gold, a luxurious green tapestry stretching into the endless horizon. An uneasy alliance existed between wild beauty and bottled tension. By day we fought, but at night we slept together, united beneath the raised benediction of the shipyard cranes.

Though I grew up in one of the most sheltered areas of Belfast, the 'Troubles', as they were known, were impossible to escape. Explosions and bomb scares were a weekly occurrence, but we were accustomed to the monotony of bag-checking, the constant army presence, the checkpoints and the border controls. Such conflict was explained in the playground long before we were taught it in the classroom. The inevitable questions: 'Where do you live?' 'What do your parents do?' 'What's your name?'

Small talk? Far from it. Your answers betrayed the fundamentals of your identity. They fixed you immovably in your place.

* * *

And so we come full circle – back to the ten-year-old me and her question, 'What's in a name?'

In some senses, nothing. Life, after all, has barely begun. As a child, I gazed expectantly ahead, into a future filled with hope and promise. My world was exciting and mysterious. Death had not yet darkened it.

Within my family, I felt secure and loved. I worked hard and did well at school. I believed myself to be special. I was many things: bright, anxious, outgoing, driven, restless. A little too intense. I was also waiting: poised to strike out and to make my own name.

But in another sense, it's already too late: I've been given my name. A tag that places me, politically, socially, culturally, personally. An indelible marker, betraying my side, my allegiance and my very nature.

It's my family, tight-knit and certain.

It's my people. Extrovert and withdrawn, loquacious and silent.

It's my homeland. Battered but unbowed, terrible and beautiful.

Before I'd done anything, these elements were in place. But adolescence brought them to the surface.

2 Resolved

Until the age of thirteen, my life felt safe, controlled and secure. Things made sense. I knew who I was. I knew where I belonged – especially within my family. Internally and externally, the boundaries were clear and consistent. But those childhood certainties were about to crumble.

What happened next? Death. Boys and sex and God. Puberty. A new home. A new school. Everything changed. Everything fell apart. This had a devastating impact on my relationships and sense of self. In fact, I would spend the next twenty years picking up the pieces.

God and death

It started in 1989 with my grandfather's death. I'd read about people dying in the news; I'd even heard bomb blasts, but they belonged to another world. This was different. This death was real. I struggled to make sense of it, waiting in vain for Granda to come back and for life to return to normal. Neither did.

It wasn't just that Granda had gone. Other things had changed too. One of the kids down the street was hit by a car, just outside my house. For a long time, he was gone. When he came back, he didn't come out to play football. He couldn't walk and he spoke funny – like he was drunk. A special bus came to take him to school, but he never seemed to see us, no matter how hard we waved.

At night I dreamt of flowers and tombstones. TV warned us about a new disease called 'AIDS' that couldn't be cured. We heard that you could catch it from toilet seats and swimming pools and needles. When you got it, it would kill you and blood would come out of your ears and eyes. The world seemed full of hidden dangers. Germs and pestilence lurked on every surface. I stopped using public toilets and started carrying soap so I could wash my hands when I went somewhere new. Nothing was safe.

What's the point?

For the first time, my parents didn't have the answers. Death was bigger than them – a problem that they couldn't fix. They couldn't protect me from it, or even themselves. Some day they too would disappear, just like Granda. Everyone would.

I searched in vain for explanations. What was the purpose in living if some day it would all end? Why were we here? Death smashed into our homes, but we tiptoed round the wreckage. Why did no-one say anything? Our loved ones were like loose change that had slipped down the back of the sofa. 'Looks like we've "lost" Great-Aunt

Ethel,' we'd remark, absent-mindedly. Adults spoke in riddles: cousin George had 'passed away'. He'd 'gone to a better place'. What place? Malta? Why didn't he write? And why couldn't we visit?

Dad bore my questions with endless patience. There was nothing to worry about, he said. When we died, we went back to the ground, where it was nice and peaceful. Everything was OK.

Though well intentioned, this did nothing to allay my fears. Dad, I concluded, had lost his mind. Nothing to worry about? Nice and peaceful? Of course it was *quiet* – you were dead! Buried alone, under layers of cold, dark earth. Death was like a horror film come true, a terrifying marauder who stole away those we cared about most. It was the epitome of Not OK.

It was clear that I would have to find the answers elsewhere. Somewhere that took death seriously and didn't tuck it under the carpet. Somewhere like church.

Up until now, I'd thought little of God. My parents weren't particularly religious, but as a child I had been baptized and went to Sunday school. In the Northern Irish context, church takes on a certain flavour. Against a backdrop of terrorism and moralism, sin and hell can seem more fitting than grace and forgiveness. Much has changed since then – and not just in my home parish. At the time, however, the preaching matched the pews – dusty, hard and uncomfortable. But what sort of God did I expect?

As a serious-minded perfectionist, my concept of God was, well, a bit like me. Except a little – bigger. He was a bearded moralist in the sky. Aloof and distant, Big and Far-Off and Right. A divine extension of teachers or parents, but far too important to notice a mixed-up girl.

In some ways, this distance was a good thing. As long as I kept my head down, he would look after his universe and I would look after mine. No interference and no mess. Never the twain need meet, right?

Not quite. At least, that's what my best friend, Deborah, argued. According to her, God knew everything about us. Worse still, he wanted 'in' on our lives – even the messy bits we tried to keep hidden. She and her family were 'Christians' and went to a Pentecostal church, where they prayed and talked to God, sometimes in a language I couldn't understand. They even played guitars! It was scandalous. But, despite myself, I was intrigued. Who was the personal God she seemed to know as a friend? What was it that made her family unique? They had the same struggles as everyone else, yet their attitude was very different and they had a certain peace. They didn't argue like us and their rules came from the Bible. Could their God also have the answers I was searching for?

I decided to investigate. Deborah invited me to a church camp, where they explained what they believed. They talked about someone called Jesus. Apparently, God had a Son. I'd heard of him already, but to these Christians he was *really* important. They were also very keen on the Bible. It wasn't a fairy story, they said, or even an ordinary book. It was written by God, and it explained how the world was made and how we should be living. But we didn't listen to God or what he said. Instead, we did what we wanted and ignored him. All of us broke his laws. This meant that we were *all* 'sinners'. And not just the murderers or paedophiles either.

I knew some of God's rules already, like telling the truth and obeying your parents. (Funnily enough, Mum and Dad had passed that one on.) Others – like listening to him – were new. I'd been breaking them for years and hadn't realized it! Sin, it seemed, was very serious. Unless we said sorry (or 'repented'), we would go to hell: a place where the fires burned forever and no-one could get out. But – and this is how my thirteen-year-old brain understood it – if I did apologize and tried my hardest to be better, then I would escape. Instead of suffering in the afterlife, I would go to heaven and live with God forever.

To me, this made sense. For one thing, it explained why I always felt so guilty. Heaven sounded a bit boring – what would we *do* all day apart from playing the harp and sitting on clouds? – but the alternative was unthinkable. There were other advantages too. Hearing about this God gave life a purpose – it meant that we were created for a reason. Somehow, wonderfully, God cared about us – including me. He promised to help me and never to leave. In some ways, I had been right all along – I *was* special. The Bible said so! Death too had an explanation and an answer. To access it, all I had to do was say a special prayer, apologizing to God for acting like he wasn't there. Instead of living according to my rules, I would now obey and follow him. It was a bit like sending off a stamped addressed envelope and getting salvation back in the post.

After I'd prayed, there was no bolt of lightning. I looked the same, but I did feel different. Relieved. Like setting down a rucksack that was filled with rocks. News spread around the camp and I became something of a celebrity: 'Emma has been saved!' Everyone was congratulating me and asking how I felt. It was a good question: I was pleased, excited, tired and emotional. But also slightly confused.

Some things remained a mystery. Who was this Jesus? And why did he die? I wasn't entirely sure. How was I supposed to 'have a relationship' with him? And where would he live? If Jesus 'came into my heart', wouldn't that hurt? And what exactly did he want?

At my home church, your mind and your will were what mattered most. You made the decision to go with God and you stuck by it, even though it was painful. In fact, that was sort of the point – proof that you were on the right path. At Deborah's church, however, the opposite seemed true. What counted there was how you felt. If you felt unhappy, then you were doing something wrong. You weren't properly 'saved'. Maybe you didn't love God as much as you should, or have enough 'faith'. Or perhaps you'd prayed 'the prayer' wrong. Either way, to be a Christian, you needed to *feel* like one.

My new-found Christianity left me relieved, but bewildered too. On Sunday mornings I got strait-laced Presbyterianism. God the Father, dry facts and church organs. Everything regimented, everything in its (right) place. On Sunday evenings I got happy-clappy Pentecostalism. The Holy Spirit, feelings and guitars. Spontaneous, messy and free-flowing.

Missing Person

As you may have spotted, something, or rather Someone, was missing. I had God the Father and God the Holy Spirit, but no Jesus. A double act instead of a Trinity. I didn't know it then, but this would have profound implications for my faith. God wanted rule-keeping and the Spirit promised feelings, but I couldn't drum up either. I just wanted him to pretend that the past stuff hadn't happened and to help me try harder.

I was confused about a lot of things. The God I followed was real and personal, and I knew he cared for me. He listened to my prayers, and I believed that the Bible was true. But, to be honest, we hadn't been properly introduced. My brand of Christianity had space for 'God', but not for Jesus. It talked about sin and rules – but less about grace. It paid lip service to his work on my behalf. But, in practice, it was up to me.

There was another problem with my new faith: my family. They hadn't been to camp. They hadn't prayed the prayer and been forgiven. This meant that they were still going to die, and much, much worse. I felt like their salvation depended on me. So I burst home, determined to persuade them of the truth.

'I'm a Christian now,' I explained. 'and you need to be too or you're going to hell.'

They couldn't see it. So I decided to show them. I did the washing up, hoovered the house and took out the rubbish – all without being asked. I ran errands, helped my brother and sister, and tried to be on my very best behaviour. I might have been the only teenager in the world whose parents told her to *stop* doing chores. It was exhausting. But I needed them to see that I was different, and this was real.

Despite my best efforts, they remained unconvinced.

'Why are you being so weird?' said my sister.

'It's a phase,' said Dad.

'That's fine for you, Emma,' said Mum, 'but it's not what we believe.'

There was no plan B, so I had to keep trying. Eternity hung in the balance. I was going to live forever – but my family were going to hell. And it was up to me to stop them.

For the first time in my life, I was different from my family. This was something new. When I had had problems in the past, there was nothing that we couldn't share. But after enduring weeks of evangelistic zeal, my parents cracked. 'This conversation is closed,' they said. 'We'll hear no more about it.' It was the beginning of a changed relationship. My parents had been my best friends – but now there were things we just couldn't discuss. I wanted their respect and their approval. I wanted to belong. Now I stuck out like a sore thumb. I had chosen to be different and I couldn't go back.

Sex, boys and my body

It wasn't just Christianity that made me different. My body was turning against me as well. Curves were spilling out, where before there had been reassuring hollows. I was terrified, but this was something else I couldn't discuss. It was embarrassing, private and shameful. Yet worse was to come. One afternoon at school, a classmate took me aside. She'd discovered something shocking: how babies were made. I listened, fascinated but aghast. How could anyone imagine something so unnatural? Impossible. Disgusting! We could no longer be friends. When Mum asked why, I burst into tears. This precipitated The Sex Talk. Next day the Usborne *Facts of Life* book appeared on my bed. Feigning indifference, I scoured its pages under cover of darkness. Yet what I discovered only worsened the situation. Suddenly I was expected to think about boys and sex and relationships. This was more than a shift in my comfort zones. It was an entirely different universe.

I was at home in a world of books. Unfazed by quests, magic, or even dragons. But this? This was gross ... unstoppable and uncontrollable. Like being strapped into a juggernaut without a seat belt. It was bigger than me – but a part of me too.

When I looked in the mirror, a stranger scowled back. She was all wrong – not a girl, but nothing like the women I saw on TV either. I still played football, but I was changing, and even the boys knew it. I saw them looking at me sometimes and whispering together. What were they saying? I was so ugly.

One of my footie friends asked me to go to the cinema with him. I was confused. What for? We saw plenty of each other every day after school. He wrote me a letter, asking if we could kiss. *With tongues*. I was revolted. Wasn't that how AIDS began? I returned the mug he'd given me, but not his calls.

Mum took me to buy a bra, but there was nothing there to fill it. I cried in the changing rooms. My old clothes didn't fit. The new ones were all wrong. There were hairs on my legs. It was like watching *The Fly*, but I couldn't stop the tape. Worse still, I was bleeding! I hadn't cut myself, but it hurt. Not just once – every single month now, for the rest of my life. Could other people tell what was happening? Surely shame was written across my face. I had to wear a nappy or, worse still, insert something inside me, something cold and painful and hard. Everyone else used tampons, so why couldn't I? Was this what sex was like? If so, I wanted no part of it.

Church youth group was full of veiled warnings about the dangers of teen pregnancies. Your body was like something separate: it would spiral out of control if you let it. Sex could take you to hell. At school you were either a virgin or a slapper – and it was hard to know which was worse. As well as AIDS, now I was afraid of getting pregnant too. I knew what the *Facts of Life* said, but you couldn't be too careful. Granny used to say we Sloans were a fertile bunch. Maybe you could get babies like flu? Every night I ran my hands across my stomach, checking for tell-tale signs. I started wearing dark, baggy clothes. I wanted to disappear, to stop people from looking at me. My body had betrayed me. It was an enemy that I couldn't control, and I hated it.

The securities I'd clung to as a child were strangling me as an adolescent. My parents and I started arguing. I was bewildered by all the changes – and I think they were too. Their little girl had been replaced by a moody teenager.

Every young person falls out with their parents. But it tore me apart. Half of me wanted to flee my old life, while half of me never wanted to grow up. While I'd previously spent hours playing with my siblings, such pursuits now seemed childish and tame. We drifted apart, though for a time my sister trailed me mutely, like a shadow. 'Go away!' I shouted. 'Get your own life!'

I longed to be left alone, for space to hide and lick my wounds. Michael hung my bras out of the window, and Ruth borrowed my clothes. We shared a room and were always arguing. I couldn't use the bathroom without someone knocking on the door. The situation was unbearable. Miraculously, Mum and Dad agreed. They told us that we were moving house – I would get my own room there and I'd be starting a new school too. There was just one problem. The new house wouldn't be ready for another three months, so we would have to live with Granny until then. Luckily, I loved Granny dearly. How difficult could it be?

Moving on

On moving day, however, I had a knot in my stomach. I paced through the rooms, stroking the walls with my fingers. I sat in the garden, one last time. Knelt by the yellow rose bush, planted on the day I was born. I thought about the hours I'd spent there, weaving and populating a private universe. I said goodbye to our old neighbours, my football buddies and the scary twins who lived down the street. Goodbye to my best friend Deborah, going to a new school. I'd passed the eleven-plus exam, but she had failed. We swore we'd keep in contact, but knew we wouldn't.

Without Granda, Granny's house felt strange. It was tiny, and the six of us were squeezed into two bedrooms. Granny was my ally, but she made a terrible bedfellow. She snored, and her talcum powder made me sneeze. There was nowhere to be alone. We did our best, but tempers got frayed, and resentments flared over the smallest things. I felt like a giant, living in a doll's house. There was far too much of me and nowhere to hide.

Three months dragged past but, when we finally moved, the new place felt cavernous and unfamiliar. Disorientated, I stalked the corridors, lost without my old friends and routine. I had threatened murder over my granny's snoring, but without her the bed seemed lonely and cold. We played cards with the boys next door, and Mum and Dad teased me about my new 'boyfriend'. He was just a mate, I protested, blushing furiously. Secretly, however, I wondered what it would feel like to kiss him – or indeed, anyone other than a blood relative. At a friend's slumber party we watched a film called *Dirty Dancing* about a gorgeous dancer who fell in love with an ordinary girl.

When he took off his shirt, something crumpled in my stomach. I kissed his poster by my bed and wore away a hole where his mouth had been. But our relationship was all in my head. I had two left feet and braces on my teeth: in real life, he would find me repulsive. Why couldn't my life match up to the films?

Moving house wasn't the only big change. I had moved from a primary co-ed to a girls' grammar school. To say that it was achievement-focused would be something of an understatement. People, I learned, were either winners or losers. Winners were smart or sporting. Preferably both. Losers tried hard, but came in second place.

I'd barely surrendered Santa Claus, but we were being urged to Consider The Future. It was impossible: I had no idea who I was, let alone what I wanted to be. The school careers computer matched my profile to that of a prison warden, while teachers suggested that I 'aim for Oxbridge'. But university was as unimaginable as Mars: I hadn't even picked my GCSEs yet.

At my old school, I was a big fish in a small pond: used to being top of the class. Now I had to prove myself all over again. I set my sights on the English prizes, agonizing over essays that burst the bounds of their staples. Maths and science were hopeless, but if I upped my game, even the needlework trophy was within reach. Strangely, however, no-one else was impressed. In a sea of apathy, my lonely hand shot up like a rocket. At first, I wore my brain on my sleeve, but when even the teachers grew weary, I learned to tuck it in my pocket instead. I decided that I would feign indifference and world-weary cynicism. This old trophy? I could take it or leave it. Though still a good student, I'd grasped an important new lesson. Being myself was not an option – unless I wanted to be slaughtered in the common room. However, this wisdom dawned a little too late.

Even today, large groups of women make me twitch. Female conventions fill me with fear – and, like Roald Dahl's witches, I'm sure they can smell it. Girls aren't straightforward, like guys. They're a mystery – and I'm supposed to be one of them. Girls hunt in packs. They never say what they mean. They smell funny and they whisper and giggle and scream – for no apparent reason. One moment they love you, and your schoolbag is simply *divine*, ohmywordwheredidyougeddit? The next, they're flushing your head down the toilet and sticking pins in your eyes. Metaphorically, at least.

I made a new best friend who was also a Christian. We were inseparable and could tell each other anything. She was from a Pentecostal background, so my models of church continued unchanged. Meanwhile the Christian Union filled more of a social than a spiritual gap. I still believed, but God was quietly but firmly relegated to Sunday services.

Among my pretty friends, I was the brainy one. But brains no longer counted. Outside school, it was a totally new social scene – boys and parties and what you wore and how you looked and whether or not your legs were smooth. However hard I shaved, I always seemed to miss a bit: the cheap razors left both my ankles and my self-esteem in shreds.

I experimented with Mum's make-up. Blue eyeshadow and orange panstick – like a Fraggle drawn with crayons. My clothes were equally wrong. Some were handed down from cousins and had been cutting edge – thirty years ago. Dad cut my hair in the style of a Franciscan monk, and I had to be home hours before all of my friends. We weren't allowed to watch the same TV shows and it felt like a language I couldn't speak. So I stuck with the language I knew best – I worked hard. And as you can probably guess, I was bullied.

The myth of 'sticks and stones' is precisely that – a poisonous lie. Words do hurt, especially when they're tossed like rocks by your peers. I felt battered already, but these daily stonings completed the process. 'You're pathetic, ugly. No-one likes you. We all hate you. Why don't you just go away and die?' I wasn't the only person to be bullied, but it shattered any confidence I had left. My parents helped me as much as they could. Night after night, Dad would sit at the end of my bed and talk me into going back to school – but he couldn't be there and he couldn't protect me. Neither could my best friend. We shared everything – but even this was sullied.

'You're a pair of lesbians!' screamed the ringleader. 'You're disgusting.'

Was she right? We were so close – perhaps that too was wrong. Maybe I was a lesbian! After all, I hadn't even had a proper boyfriend. I felt confused and ashamed.

'We can't be friends any more,' I said. 'I need some space.'

The bullies found new targets, but I became lonely and isolated. I still worked hard, but the plaudits meant little and I mocked the teachers I had previously adored. I pretended I had a cloak that made me invisible and shielded me from others. Perhaps the answer was to make myself smaller and act like everything was OK. So I tacked on a smile and ate my lunch alone. I prayed to God to help me, but every day my self-hatred grew. It became clear that I would have to rescue myself. The old me wasn't working: time to make a new one.

Masks

I began by adopting a fresh persona – as class joker. While previously I had played it safe and blended in, now I became loud and reckless instead. My waking hours were spent inventing quips and planning new ways to entertain, always at my own expense. I affected a detachment to opinion and regaled my classmates with tall stories. Internally, however, I was in an agony of vigilance, measuring every word for its effect. I no longer knew who I was. All that mattered were the reflections mirrored back at me by my peers. Despite their laughter, I felt that they secretly despised me. How could they not? I slipped on bravado like my uniform, then left it bundled in a heap on the floor. Perhaps some traces of the old me remained, but she was unspeakably, obscenely ugly. I wanted her dead.

In one sense, my world was closing down. I wanted more emotional and physical space, but I had less. It was too small and too tight, and I just couldn't breathe. Yet in another sense, the world was also opening out. I felt overwhelmed by change, internal and external: constantly divided and pulled in opposing directions. Part of me wanted to embrace the future and set forth boldly towards a new horizon. The rest wanted to curl up like a comma, to hide and never grow up.

I knew that God was there but didn't believe he could care for me – after all, even my family found me annoying and I had no real friends. At youth group I stuck out like a sore thumb: I was the only person from a non-Christian background and, in case they forgot, I kept blurting out blasphemous mistakes. The safest solution was to stop asking questions and keep very still. In the talks they said that God loved everyone, but in practice they ignored me and I was never invited to their parties. After months of pleading, one morning Mum accompanied me to church. No-one said hello, and we were asked to move three times because the pews were 'kept for regulars'. Humiliated, we left early and it was years before we returned.

All I wanted was to fit in. I didn't feel like a Christian, and being religious was just another way of standing out. God, I decided, was just like all the rest – interested in what I did, not who I was.

Every day I donned a new mask and every night I tumbled into bed, defeated and depressed. I hated my life and I hated my neediness: this insatiable longing to be accepted. Church, home and school were governed by an etiquette I could neither see nor understand. My head hurt from trying to make sense of it.

'Work hard. Lighten up. Stand out. Fit in. Don't just go with the crowd, but don't attract attention to yourself either. Do well at school, but not too well – and never, ever look like you're trying.'

'It's what's on the inside that matters. But if you're not wearing Nikes, you're better off dead.'

'You're special. You're a freak. Be yourself – but listen to the critics. Honour your parents, but don't let them baby you.'

'Grow up! You're still a minor. Start thinking for yourself! When you're under our roof, missy, you'll obey our rules.'

'Speak up. Simmer down. Work out what you're doing with your life. Don't take everything so seriously.'

'Feel the love. Jesus wants you for a sunbeam. Onward, Christian soldier! Suffering now, glory later.

God so loves the world that whosoever keeps his rules
will never perish. Remember, Emma, it's all about
grace.'
'Get a boyfriend. Get experience. You're frigid. You're
a whore.'
'You're invisible. You take up too much space. No-one
listens to what you say. How can anyone take you
seriously? You're attention-seeking. Don't be shy.
Listen, young lady, the world doesn't revolve around
you.'

On the outside, the wheels kept turning. Internally, however, I was grinding to a halt. I lacked the energy to keep
pretending – not to my family, not to my teachers, not to
my classmates and not to God. But what was the
alternative?

'School days,' opined the grown-ups, 'are the happiest
days of your life.' They had to be joking. Death had been
my greatest fear, but if life looked like this, it was a
stinking lie.

One day I caught sight of my reflection and something
in me snapped. As I looked in the mirror, I saw myself as
if for the first time: a nerd who'd lost her childhood,
petrified of adolescence, confused and Christian, bullied,
isolated, unsure of what it meant to be a woman, and
wrenched in a hundred different directions. Worst of all,
I was completely, terrifyingly, out of control. In that
moment, I made a decision. Whatever the cost, I would
take control back.

This was how my anorexia began.

3 Relentless

Where does anorexia come from – and what is it? There are, I suspect, a thousand answers. It's bullying, Barbie and biology. It's sickness and it's sin. It's death and God and the universe. It's 'us' and it's 'them'. It's global media and the kitchen table. It's the Western world and it's the human heart.

In my case, it was a thirteen-year-old with a particular type of personality. Perfectionistic. Obsessive. Insecure. Bright. Intense.

What else?

A close-knit family, struggling to let go.

A place, filled with banter and bombs.

A people, charged with passion, but frightened of emotion.

A culture, where individuality and conformity collide.

A church, struggling to be in, but not of, 'the world'.

A time of life when body and circumstances are changing.

And last but not least, a human heart determined to have its own way.

Brand 'Nice'

I've always striven to be one of life's 'good' girls. I want to fit. This rules out certain avenues of rebellion – like drink, drugs or sex. (Sorry to disappoint. I must warn you, there are no 'love rats' or car chases in this book either.)

Put bluntly, I was an approval-seeking missile. Someone who kept the rules, ticked the right boxes and respected authority. Someone who craved acceptance – from grown-ups, peers, small children and even animals. Someone for whom the word 'Nice' meant more than a brand of biscuit. 'Nice' was my brand: pastel-coloured, vanilla-flavoured and inoffensive. Being 'Nice' allowed me to fly under the radar. I might not have been popular, but I hoped I'd be safe. Nice girls are prefects – or, like me, deputy head girl. We have the grades for the top job, but not quite the charisma.

Everyone knows young people like this. The 'perfect' child, the earnest student. Stalwart of the Bible study, always ready with the 'right' answers ('Jesus' is usually a safe bet). The ones who never seem to do anything wrong. Who can be relied upon to stay the course, toe the line and return their library books well within the deadlines. The ones who never give anyone any trouble. But maybe this is part of the problem. Troublemakers tend to get the most attention. Good girls soldier on and seem stable, but their pristine exteriors can mask all kinds of issues. Left unnoticed, these may bubble away for years. Yet the eruption, when it comes, can be spectacular.

As someone who depends upon order, 'going off the rails' is not an option. You're much too scared to take risks or make any mess. When even an unmade bed feels threatening, sex and drugs hold little appeal. You're not seeking the bad stuff 'out there'. You fear the bad stuff 'in here' – underneath your skin.

When adolescence hits, the good girl won't 'break out'. But she might well break down. Quietly, of course.

Growing pains

Adolescence was, for me, an unparalleled trauma. My teenage body felt messy and chaotic: everything seemed to be bursting its banks. Feelings and fears were multiplied to extremes. It was far more than I could cope with.

I kept a journal, but was terrified that someone would read it. The person reflected in its pages disgusted me, and so I burned it in the garden. My English essays still scored well, but they became increasingly dark, splattered with blood and self-hatred. Teachers put it down to an overactive imagination and too many gothic novels. They didn't know that I was toiling through the night, obsessively reworking my scripts. For a GCSE geography project I spent three days, locked in my room, drawing and colouring an intricate map of Ireland. When I made a tiny mistake, I threw it away and started again. No matter what I did, it wasn't good enough. My grades were all that I had left – I couldn't afford to lose those too.

I was afraid of almost everything. Public toilets, covered in germs. AIDS and terrorism. Boys, babies and sex. For my family, dying and heading for hell. Only I could stop them, but they wouldn't listen. My anxieties grew worse.

What if people could read my thoughts? Or if I shouted something obscene in the street? My words came out all wrong, and I was sick of making mistakes.

I withdrew from friends and social occasions. I had to protect myself. I had to protect those I loved. I watched my brother playing in the street. What if he was hit by a car? How would I rescue him? Perhaps I could earn his safety and buy him a little more time. If I chanted the alphabet backwards, he might be OK.

I started developing little routines, patterns that shielded me from the outside world. Checking over what I'd written, three, four or even five times. As a child, I was fascinated by magic: I pretended to be a sorceress and warded off evil by filling scrapbooks with 'spells'. As a teenager, I created new rituals to do the same job. Everything had to be counted. The steps from the toilet to the kitchen. The pages of my textbooks. Stripes on the wallpaper. Carbohydrates in a milkshake. The calories in a piece of cheese.

I searched food labels for answers, like a fortune-teller scouring tea leaves. Seeking a name for what I was feeling and a reason for what was wrong. I memorized the breakdown of each item until I didn't need to look. And in the packaging I found something else. I discovered myself. There was a label for my ugliness and my mess. A name for all that had changed and gone wrong in my life.

'Fat.'

I was fat.

Feelings and food

Growing up, there were no issues of weight in my family. I was teased for wearing 'trainer bras' and we rehearsed the standard jokes about my bum causing a solar eclipse. However, my comic 'timing', chicken walk and total lack of common sense were just as fruitful. That's siblings, that's school and that's life. I gave back as good as I got. But at home at least, I felt no pressure about my size.

Mealtimes were a focus in our house. Amid the busyness of the day, it was at the kitchen table that our family would regroup. We sat in the same seats and ate in the same order – Dad at the head, always served first. Dinner tended to be typical Irish fare – meat and two veg. We didn't have sweets, but made up for it by plundering the fruit bowl and the fridge. Even today it's a running joke that at breakfast we'll start thinking about lunch and at lunch we'll be talking about dinner.

This, however, is a global as well as a local preoccupation. Our culture tells us to spoil ourselves – then reminds us that thin is 'in'. From the earliest age, we're taught to have our cake – but not to eat it.

I began to think about the relationship between what I ate and who I was:

I thought about the child that I had left behind and the woman I was becoming. Frightened of the future, but locked out of the past.

I thought about my body. Post-puberty, it stopped being my own. Now it was something separate, alien and even threatening. It no longer did what it was told. Physically and emotionally, it overflowed.

I thought about no longer fitting into my old clothes. And not fitting in – at school, at church or at home.

I thought about my stomach, curved instead of concave. The bits that should have stuck out but didn't, and the bits that stuck out but should have stayed hidden.

I thought about my ideals. The women in the stories that I loved: pale and consumptive, feminine and frail. The heroic saints, fasting in godly isolation, far removed from the chaotic desires of body and world. I thought about the older girls at school, exotic and aloof, always in a crowd. Always on a diet.

I thought about my family, sitting around the dinner table. The pains of negotiating adulthood. Our arguments. The constant battles – about who I saw and where I went. Sitting at the table till I'd swallowed my food and accepted my place. The anger and the frustration, burning in my throat.

I thought about my hungers. The ways I ought to have been different and the ways that I already was. About being invisible and unseen, but also too intense and too much. About my appetites and the suspicion that they could never be met. The loneliness of the school canteen. The fear that I would spend my whole life feeling hungry.

I thought and I thought and I thought. But I reached no conclusions.

* * *

Life went on, but the future started to encroach upon the present. We had to choose our GCSEs, and I opted for home economics – food studies. I was a good student and became fascinated by diet and sustenance. I swapped my novels for cookbooks and entered a national competition called: 'Young Cook of the Year'. I even made it to the finals, with an inspired combination of tuna and banana, entitled 'Spicy Brunchy Balls'. Its glycaemic index was flawless, but the taste left much to be desired.

Nutrition was soothing – it could be arranged into neat boxes: carbohydrates, fats, proteins, fibres. Even within these groups, there were subdivisions, clearly marked and designated. For the curious, they opened up a strange and fascinating alchemy. Proteins could be separated into high-biological and low-biological values. But when you mixed two of the lesser ones, you got the whole package. Iron was hard to absorb on its own, but when you mixed it with vitamin C – presto! Your body drank it down.

Every day, mysterious processes were going on within us. My own metamorphosis made this painfully clear. Now I knew why. I'd finally found a bit of biology I could understand – a chemistry that I could control. It worked like this: what you put in showed up on your body – in your skin, your teeth, even your brain. This might appear obvious, but to me it was a revelation. More than this, it seemed to be the answer I was looking for. Food was *it*. An explanation. An obsession. An addiction. Hiding it. Cutting it back. Whittling down the 'safe' items, one by one . . . until I was eating hardly anything at all.

'Fat'

Like many addictions, this one started small. I remember one afternoon in late summer. It had been a long day, and we'd had a double session of physical education, which I hated. Regulation 'sportswear' was a tiny cotton vest and 'forest green' nappies which doubled as woollen knickers. Amid the clouds of body spray and talc, we would furtively assess one another, the louder girls preening like peacocks and parading their cleavage. The bullies were brilliant at sports and, while the classroom offered some sanctuary, this was their undisputed domain.

Innuendo and insults flew across the locker room like missiles. Dressed in mismatched (grey) trainer bra and pants, I was an easy target.

Sometimes we did aerobics in the lunch hall. The floor was covered in a thin layer of dust and smelt of ham sandwiches and feet. As the pretty girls high-kicked to the right, I would unerringly veer left, seven steps behind and always missing the beat. The alternative was swimming, which was even worse. We used the pool at a nearby boys' school and were herded like cattle past mobs of jeering youths. Then the fun began in earnest. The main pool was surrounded by an enormous spectators' gallery and glass panels which opened out onto the sports field. To reach it, you had to negotiate your way through a disinfectant footbath: 2 inches of putrid water, studded with plasters and pubic hairs. One week a girl threw up in it, and we had to pick our way through bits of sweetcorn instead. Once in the gallery, we would huddle by the side of the pool, trying to fold ourselves into tiny triangles. I begged Mum for a sick note citing Ebola or jungle fever – anything to escape the boys and the footbath.

On this particular day, we were neither swimming nor high-kicking.

'Good news, girls!' boomed the gym teacher. 'It's fitness testing week.'

Our first challenge was to outrun a machine emitting an increasingly insistent 'bleep'. You started by sprinting across the grass pitch and, each time it bleeped, you had to turn round and run back. The machine started ridiculously fast and sped up from there. Just looking at it was exhausting, and we lost some girls to detention for 'bleeping' along with it. Clutching our bellies, we dropped like flies by the side of the track and, ever the champion,

I led the fall-out. But there was more to come. 'Let's test your body fat!' bellowed Trunchbull, furiously blowing her whistle.

Filing obediently back to the changing rooms, we were stripped to our underwear, and then weighed. In full view of our classmates. A tape measure was wrapped across our chests, and the results recorded in a blue plastic file. Then the nurse produced an enormous pair of callipers.

'Lift up your shirt,' she said. 'And stop breathing in.'

The plastic pincers stretched and measured how fat we were – our arms, thighs and stomachs. It was disgusting, but there was nowhere to hide. I wanted to die. In the common room afterwards, lunches remained untouched, and even the non-smokers decamped to the bus shelter. In class we giggled nervously and passed around articles about Wonderbras and diets.

That afternoon I slunk home and pulled on my tracksuit. The waistband dug in and, when I leant forward, I could still grab the excess flesh. Pure fat. Gross.

Dad rang the dinner bell, and I went downstairs to join my family at the kitchen table.

'Good day?' asked Mum.

'Smashing,' I said.

Conversation washed around me as I picked at my food. Meat, veg, potatoes. I sliced the potatoes in half and asked Mum to pass me the butter. As my knife cut into the yellow spread, I paused. Then a light went on. This was the problem. Fat.

I took a breath and slowly, carefully replaced the butter lid.

'I'm not very hungry,' I said. 'In fact, I feel a bit sick.'

I pushed my chair back from the table. Lifted my plate

and scraped the remains into the bin. Then I walked away, from the kitchen and my family.

A tiny step that changed everything.

Cutting down

Little by little, I reduced what I ate. First, the fats. No more butter. No more cream. No more biscuits. I cut the corners of my lamb chops, pushed my chips to the side, feigned fullness. I watched, exhilarated, as the scales grew lighter.

Next came carbohydrates. Potatoes, rice, pasta. I would find excuses for not eating:

'I've had dinner already.'
'I'm really stuffed.'
'This Bolognese tastes funny.'
'I'll eat later.'

Mum and Dad weren't happy. They usually tried to make me finish, but occasionally let it pass. I skipped breakfast, racing out the door before I had time to be questioned. Or I'd flourish some toast, before secretly tossing it, along with lunch, into the bin. Even at school no-one asked any questions. Lots of girls skipped lunch. Lots of girls were on a diet.

Proteins were next to go: 'I think I'd like to be a vegetarian.'

Dad snorted, and I knew better than to argue. Undeterred, I cut up my chicken and hid it under the vegetables, in my pockets, or my shoes. I smuggled it into napkins, or up my sleeves. I chewed and spat food into my drinks or even onto the floor. I poured hot chocolate (my 'favourite') into the plants and pleaded ignorance when they died. This was before the internet took off – but women's magazines already provided a fund of new knowledge. 'When you're cold, you burn off calories,' they said. I lay on my bed with the windows open, shivering in my soaking underwear. It was worth it: my waistband no longer chafed. In fact, it grew looser. Finally, I had to pin it together.

Guilty secret

With practice, I grew better at hiding the evidence. This was my secret, and it was vital that no-one suspect. I behaved like a fugitive, disguising my tracks. I became adept at hiding, lying and pretending that nothing had changed. I wore dark, baggy clothes, always with pockets. I invented cinema trips, but went for long walks instead. At lunchtimes I would run around the sports field. I discovered an old Jane Fonda book of aerobics and practised stomach crunches, star-jumps and press-ups in my room. Every day I added more, until I was exercising for hours at a time, often through the night. Muscles started to develop beneath the skin. More thrilling still, I could feel my bones jutting through the fabric. I was getting my old body back. Even my dreaded periods grew lighter – then stopped. But there was still a long way to go. As I reached a new goal weight, the number always dropped. Just a little more. Push a little harder. I ran to and from school, even in the rain. And the more I exercised, the less I ate.

Bit by bit, the 'safe' foods shrank. Fruit and vegetables became dangerous. I licked foods guiltily, then spat them out. Fearful of the calories in toothpaste, I stopped cleaning my teeth. Every morning and evening I balanced excitedly on the scales, watching with fascination as the numbers dropped. And as this passion grew, others waned. My brain wasn't quite as sharp as it had once been. It felt fuzzy and disconnected. To achieve the same grades, I now had to work much harder. Sometimes I would read the same page, over and over, before the words sank in. When I stood up too quickly, I felt sick and dizzy. But none of this mattered. Light-headed and tight-lipped, I crested a wave of private exultation.

I stopped going out. I didn't want to see anyone – friends, family, even Granny. The things I had once cared about no longer seemed important. Even if people hated me, I didn't care. Let them whisper – now I was beyond their reach and they couldn't hurt me. I had a secret they knew nothing about, something they couldn't control. My body was mine and mine alone. It made me powerful and untouchable. The more I shrank it, the stronger I became.

Yet as I lost more and more weight, my skeleton became harder to hide. The first person to notice was the girl who had bullied me at school. She had found a new target, but I no longer cared. One day she pulled me aside in the corridor.

'You've gotten very thin,' she said. 'Are you all right?'

I thanked her warmly for her concern. She could go to hell. They all could. *Now* I was getting noticed by the popular girls. *Now* they wanted to be my friend. As the pounds dropped off, I gloried in their envy.

'I wish I was as skinny as you,' they said. 'I wish I had your self-control.'

At home, however, it was a different story. Dinner with

my parents was impossible to avoid. The table had become a battleground – and the good girl, a rebel.

Family outings were excruciating too. I trailed several steps behind, morose and angry, a wraith wearing headphones. My parents grew worried, frustrated and finally angry.

'What's wrong with you?' they asked.

'I'm fine!' I howled back, barricading myself in my bedroom. 'Just leave me alone!'

'You're so weird,' hissed my brother. Even my sister withdrew and made her own friends.

'Why can't you cheer up and start acting normal?' said Dad.

They didn't understand. But truth be told, neither did I.

The descent

Anorexia doesn't happen overnight. It's often slow, insidious and imperceptible. However, once started, it's like a juggernaut, gaining its own relentless momentum.

One of my friends has a black Labrador, and we used to take him for walks in the park. Sometimes we'd throw the ball and he would run down the hill after it. He'd start off at a gentle pace but, as the incline grew steeper, he would be forced to gather speed. Bewildered, he was unable to stop, no matter how hard he tried. He would overshoot the ball and come crashing to a standstill, usually aided by a tree. We would bandage him up, but next week he would do the same thing again.

Eating disorders can be similar. You start with an achievable aim in mind. Maybe to 'just lose a few pounds'. Or 'fit into that skirt, in time for the wedding'. You set off at a gentle canter. But as the goal approaches, you gather speed. You're racing past the initial target, but at first it doesn't matter. The big day passes and you're high on compliments. The skirt's too big, but you can't stop now – your adrenalin is pumping and you're moving faster and faster. The world starts to become a bit of a blur. You're lost in the chase.

By the time you spot the tree ahead, it's already too late. People around you shout warnings, but they're too far off and you can't really hear them. What started as a game has become something darker, and you can't stop, even if you want to. Your body is a rocket, propelling itself forwards. *If* you will crash is no longer in question. It's whether or not you'll get back up.

The whirlpool effect

When your weight falls below a certain threshold, it's not just your bum that shrinks. Your heart (a muscle) also wastes away. As your starved brain struggles to adjust, concentration, judgment and comprehension break down. Day by day, the disorder gathers speed. You're experiencing the 'whirlpool'.

This 'whirlpool effect' was shown powerfully in 'The Minnesota Starvation Experiment'.[2] In 1944–5, thirty-six volunteers went through a period of prolonged semi-starvation. The volunteers suffered significant increases in depression, hysteria and hypochondria. They began as healthy men, without food or body issues. Yet as the study progressed, most experienced periods of severe emotional distress and depression, including self-mutilation. They became obsessed with food, both during starvation and rehabilitation. They also reported depression, social isolation, mood swings, irritability and paranoia. One subject even amputated three fingers of his hand with an axe, though he was unsure if he had done so intentionally or accidentally.

These men had no prior difficulties with food or body image. But when their weight was anorexic, so was their thinking. The two are mutually reinforcing, and this is how the whirlpool begins. What starts as a choice becomes a tyranny instead. You think you're in charge, but you're not. That's partly because the 'you' who first embarked on this journey no longer exists. You're too far gone to see it. And even when you do, the realization can come too late.

Anorexia is, statistically, the most deadly of mental illnesses. But very few anorexics start with death as their end goal. If you want to end your life, there are quicker and easier ways of doing it. Instead, 'life' is what the disorder promises. Death, you see, is just a side effect.

Remaking my world

Puberty for me was a declaration of war, but the 'enemy' wasn't outside the gates. It was an internal insurrection. Dangerous emotions that wouldn't be silenced, a mutiny of hormones leaking out from every pore. They're bigger than you, and stronger too. If you let them escape, they'll devour you and everyone in their path.

You know this, so you swallow them and you smother them and you try to contain them. You stamp on them and you crush them and you drown them. But, like blood seeping under a closed door, they keep coming back.

I felt like a shambles: a spreading, leaking pool of weakness and need. A human spill, like red wine bleeding into a white carpet. It was unbearable. Whatever the cost, I had to soak up the mess.

So I did. By starving myself, I made myself clean. Instead of having lots of worries I couldn't manage, life became very simple. Controllable. With my body, I was able to create my own universe. A realm where I ruled, with unquestioned sovereignty. I was no longer at the mercy of my feelings. I was in charge: a self-created, stainless-steel person. Bleached to perfection. Clean and clinical and shiny and hard.

A living contradiction

The Bible says,

> There is a way that seems right to a man,
>   but in the end it leads to death.
> (Proverbs 14:12)

This is exactly right. The problem is, it feels like life. It feels magnificent.

And it works. Well, for a bit. But it's a mass of contradictions as well.

The universe is out of control, yet you're trying to mastermind everything in it. You believe you're in charge, yet you're really enslaved. The deeper you spiral down, the more you resemble what you're trying to escape.

You were the girl who was never any trouble to anyone – now you're a terrorist, and your body's the grenade that'll blow your family apart.

On one hand you're screaming out, writing over your body what you can't say with words. On the other, you're trying desperately to cover it all up.

You've got this glorious, awful secret that's bigger than you. You *want* people to help – but you'll die if they do.

You've been reborn. From the good girl who meets everyone's expectations, to a creature who'll kill anything in its way.

And God or your parents or your friends or teachers or youth leaders can all go to hell.

Anger management

At one point I told a teacher I was feeling depressed. Her response? 'Don't be ridiculous; teenagers don't get depressed.' But if hating yourself and wanting to die isn't depression, then I'm not sure what is. And if no-one else can see it, then there's only one conclusion: either the world is crazy, or you are.

Maybe 'depression' is the wrong word. Some psychologists call it 'frozen rage'. This rings true with my experience. I was not just angry. I was furious. Good girls often are.

Depression can be cold, empty and watery. It renders you helpless, immobile and pathetic. *Anger* feels very different. It's hot and sticky, concentrated and full. It propels you forwards. With anger, you can *do* something. It is energizing. It gives you a target, a scapegoat (even if it's yourself). Instead of a victim, you become an aggressor. For 'nice' girls in particular, that's seductive, but dangerous.

Covering up

How did I manage to continue this way for so long? Simple: I lied. About anything and everything. What I was doing, how I was feeling, where I'd been, what I ate. For every question, I had an answer – a paper smile and a volley of excuses. I denied that anything was wrong. I hid myself where no-one would find me: behind an impenetrable fortress of deceit and rage.

On one level, I had no idea what was happening to me. I'd never even heard of eating disorders, let alone anorexia. Yet I also knew that I was changed. I'd unleashed something wonderful, but terrible too. I might destroy myself, but I would do it *my way*. Nothing and no-one would stop me. If I'm truly honest, however, there was a part of me that was scared as well.

Getting help

In a moment of rare weakness, I confided in my mum.

'I'm not feeling well,' I said. 'A bit tired. Maybe I should go to the doctor.'

She hugged me and we went. There was a long queue in the surgery, and the doctor seemed weary and distracted. I tried to explain what was wrong, but the words wouldn't come. I didn't understand it myself.

'I'm feeling a bit funny. A bit down. And not very . . . hungry.'

The doctor raised an eyebrow. He shared my teacher's view that kids didn't get depressed. 'You probably need to get out more. Are you getting enough exercise?'

Perhaps he had a point. Note to self: Redouble the jogging.

Mum folded her arms. 'We're really quite worried. It's not like her – she's not been herself. She's not sleeping and she looks thinner too. Could you examine her? Maybe check her pulse?'

He glanced at the clock again and sighed. Then he rolled up my sleeve. 'Not much of you, is there? I take it you're eating enough?'

I mumbled something, but he nodded before I'd finished.

After taking my blood pressure he turned back to Mum. 'It's low, but nothing to worry about. Look, she's a teenager. Her body's changing and it's not unusual to have irregular periods. Nothing a good night's sleep and some exercise won't sort.'

And that was that.

Fast-forward four months:

I was starving.

The dizziness had become a lot worse.

I had chest pains.

My body was covered in a thin layer of downy hair.

My ankles and wrists were swollen.

I was exhausted. I was exercising frantically but, even when I stopped, I couldn't sleep. So I would get up and do stomach crunches instead.

My periods hadn't returned.

I couldn't think. I couldn't follow conversations, headlines or a single train of thought. It was like swimming underwater. My brain was wrapped in cotton wool. The outside world was a shadow – insubstantial, dreamlike, distant. Nothing was real. All that mattered was losing weight.

I dreamt about chocolate, cheese, potatoes, butter. I awoke to the taste of terror and ran to the bathroom to rinse out my mouth. At night I ran my fingers back and forth across my ribs, counting, checking that I hadn't put on weight. I couldn't sit down because my tail bone hurt – but it still wasn't enough. I had to lose more.

I could barely speak, let alone work. My cheeks were sunken, and I was permanently cold. People were noticing that something was wrong. But I no longer cared.

Mum dismissed my objections and made an emergency appointment with another doctor. I lay silently on her couch as she probed me with her fingers. She looked worried. Made a phone call. Then another. I was told to wait outside. I tore my hanky into tiny shreds and watched listlessly as it fluttered to the floor.

They called me back in. Mum was grey and wouldn't meet my eyes.

'You're very sick,' said the doctor. 'We need to get you treatment.'

'Fine,' I mumbled. 'But I've got an assignment due in tomorrow. We can come back next week.'

The doctor paused, looked at Mum and then back at me.

'You need treatment now,' she said. 'In another week it'll be too late.'

4 Ruled

From this point onwards, things moved very fast. The house was filled with hushed discussions, conversations that stopped when I entered the room. The phone kept ringing. My brother and sister treated me differently, like I would break if they spoke. Mum and Dad were white-faced and tight-lipped. It was going to be OK, they said. Life would soon return to normal. We were getting help, and the experts would tell us what to do.

But it wasn't that simple.

We were given an emergency referral to a young people's unit in Belfast. The centre dealt with different mental health issues, and it was permanently over-subscribed. This was the early 1990s, and eating disorders were bizarre and exotic, especially in Northern Ireland. Sufferers were strangers like the late American singer Karen Carpenter or lipsticked celebrities from another planet. We were familiar with hunger strikers, but they were mentioned in hushed tones. How could such violence have smashed into the sanctuary of *our* home? It was impossible, a nightmare from which we would surely awake.

Reality bites

The young people's 'unit' was a converted flat in town. On our arrival, the buzzer was broken, so we knocked instead. Part-residential, part-outpatient, the first floor resembled a student bedsit – but with bars on the windows. There was a hole in the door, and the walls were damp and peeling. It was difficult to distinguish between staff and patients: everyone looked exhausted and grim-faced.

Straight-backed and buttoned up, we waited for the specialists to confirm their mistake. We didn't belong here; surely they would see that? The place stank of cigarettes, stale coffee and human misery. Across the hallway, we could hear screaming, crying and cursing. Mum shifted in the plastic chair. Someone turned up the television, and a door slammed.

None of this was real. None of it could touch us.

A young woman came into the hall, arms folded round a slim brown file. 'Mr and Mrs Sloan? And you must be Emma. Come on through.'

We followed her mutely, up the stairs. Past the other parents, staring blankly into space.

'Sorry, it's a bit crazy here, as usual.'

Mum winced, stretching her lips into a smile.

'Now, I just need to examine you, Emma. If you take your clothes off and lie down on the bed, I'll come back in a minute. You can keep your underwear on.'

The door closed, and I started peeling off the layers. Three jumpers. Two cardigans. Four T-shirts. Tracksuit. Four pairs of leggings. It was spring, but I was always freezing. And I couldn't show how I really looked.

I curled up on the bed, shivering under the thin sheet. My bones dug into the mattress, but the pain was reassuring, a reminder of how far I'd come. I squeezed the outline of my stomach, disgusted by the pale, dimpled flesh. Perhaps it was slightly less obvious, but I could feel the fat, pulsating under my skin. I had exercised through the night, but missed my morning walk. Later I would work twice as hard to make up for it.

The door opened, and the girl returned. She didn't seem much older than me. I wondered what she was thinking.

She asked me to stand up and weighed me – but the scales were funny. The screen was hidden, and I couldn't read what it said. It didn't matter – I knew the numbers to the very last digit. I tried to make conversation, but her lips were drawn in a tight line and she wouldn't meet my eyes. I asked if I could put my clothes back on, but she didn't answer. Instead, she opened the door and called my mum.

'I think you need to see this,' she said.

Mum looked at me, just for a second, and then turned away. Her hand flew to her throat and she made a small, choking noise.

'I'm sorry,' said the girl. 'This must be quite a shock.'

I couldn't see Mum's face, but her fingers were plucking at an invisible piece of thread. We watched as she tugged on her sleeves. Still no-one spoke. The girl led her into another room, and I started to dress, before waiting in the corridor. In the distance, a clock beat rhythmically against the wall. I tried to follow the hands as they marked out the minutes, but it was hard to stay focused. It had been at least an hour since I last exercised.

Mum and Dad returned, and dazed, we stumbled outside. Mum's eyes were red and she was shaking. She wouldn't look at me. We got back into the car and she hesitated for a moment before grabbing my hand.

'We're going to get through this, Emma,' she said. 'We're going to get you better.' I looked down. Her fingers had left red indents on my skin. She shook her head. 'I just can't believe it. You look . . . You look . . . '

It scared me to see her like this, bent over the wheel.

'Mum,' I said. 'It's going to be OK.'

She flinched, then straightened. 'Yes. It will. Of course it will.' A pause. 'It has to be.'

When we got home, Dad went to hug me, but I pulled away. I didn't like to be touched. They went into the living room, and I watched as Mum crumpled into his arms. Before the door closed, I could hear her stammering.

'Stanton, you want to see her. Like someone in a con- centration camp.' Her shoulders were heaving. 'Anorexia. That's what she's got. She's anorexic.'

Another name

Anorexia. I rolled the word around my mouth, but it felt spiky and ugly. I wanted to spit it back out. We'd heard about it in home economics. Some of the magazines mentioned it. But I'd never known anyone who actually had it. Was it a disease – like flu? And could it be cured?

As I exercised in my room, my head buzzed with questions. The ritual was always the same. Legs, arms, stomach, bum. Press-ups. Forty-one, forty-two . . . (or was it forty-three? *Start again, just to be sure*). What had I done? I was confused and anxious, but also strangely relieved. (Sixty-five, sixty-six, and another thirty . . .) I wanted to be helped, but I didn't know how. What was happening? Something dark had swallowed me and given me its name. Anorexia. I was *anorexic*.

* * *

The following weeks were a blur. Perhaps I blocked them out. But I knew one thing. I'd introduced something terrible – a poison – into our family. It was powerful and dangerous. Like me, it should have been contained.

I wanted to make things right, but I couldn't, wouldn't eat. I wanted to curl up in my father's arms and sleep there forever. To hug my mum, and never let her go. But putting on weight? Impossible. So I howled until my throat bled. I scratched and ripped and tore at anyone who came close. I cried until the tears dried up. They were threatening the only thing that gave my life meaning. Without it, I was no-one.

But I had no alternative. Adults sanctioned and circumscribed every area of my life. I was a minor, speechless and invisible.

Finish your plate

We were sent to a dietician so I could learn about nutrition.

'Fats,' she said earnestly, 'are part of a healthy, balanced diet.'

I grimaced and nodded. 'Really? I had no idea.'

Desperate to fix the situation, I volunteered to eat Mars bars for breakfast. Yet, in practice, even a crust of bread would send me spiralling into an agony of remorse and self-contempt.

My new food regime was pinned up on the kitchen wall. It was horrific. From eating hardly anything, life became one interminable mealtime. It felt like food was every-where. Breakfast, lunch, dinner. Snacks every half-hour. Biscuits. Horlicks with full-fat milk. Cheese. Potatoes. Chicken *with the skin on*. Worse still, I couldn't work it off. I was constantly being watched – even at night.

All exercise – including the short walk to the garage – was strictly forbidden. At school I wasn't allowed to go to the toilet on my own. My friends became my jailers, and I had to sit with a teacher at lunch and break-time. We pretended I was doing extra study, but everyone knew. The other girls swapped diet tips and watched me with a mixture of pity and disgust.

The situation at home was even worse. Me versus The Family. Conversation was impossible. Instead, we ranted, screamed, fought and cried. Mealtimes were a battleground, with campaigns lasting hours at a time. Once allies, we had now become sworn enemies. We plotted against each other, devising fresh strategies to break the endless stalemates. On both sides, lines were drawn and then crossed. Mum tried to smuggle butter into my food, breaching the terms of the meal plan. Hysterical, I hit my head against the wall and pushed away the plate. They pushed it back. I smuggled food up my sleeves and spat it into my coffee. They checked my pockets and replaced the mugs and bowls with clear glass. I roared and raged but, stony-faced, they held their ground. Every evening we retreated, bloodied and exhausted, to the blessed oblivion of sleep. But the morning brought with it breakfast – and a new day of conflict.

Nothing would change. I was made of steel: *I would not eat*. But my parents were immovable too. Iron met iron, and neither fork, nor will, would concede.

Retreat

In the end though, I was outmanoeuvred and out-numbered. Despite my efforts, I began to gain weight – though it was two steps forwards and one step back. We dreaded the weekly weigh-in. The day before, I would panic, fearing I'd have lost or gained weight. Either prospect was horrendous.

While I was terrified of weight gain, part of me did want to get better. I longed to redress the hurt I had caused. Sometimes I prayed, asking for extra help or confessing to fresh stratagems. But in the end I turned inwards. God was on my parents' side. He was an extension of the adults, disgusted and disappointed by my behaviour. Once I was better, we could start again. Until then, we had nothing left to say to each other.

Cracks in the foundations

As the days turned into months and my rebellion continued, my family hardened and broke. Mum and Dad started arguing. Ruth begged Mum to let her move in with Granny.

In a family that prized truth, I had broken the ultimate taboo. I was a liar, a stranger who could no longer be trusted. They loved me, but they hated what I was doing. So much for the good girl who'd never been any trouble. A furious revolutionary had taken her place.

In the history of our family, it was – and is – an agonizing chapter. Words said on both sides have left indelible marks. We've talked about it since, but there are some parts that I can't narrate. I can speak only from my perspective, and even that is flawed. There are many, many things that I don't know. Feelings I can't even guess at.

I don't know how it feels to watch, helpless, as your beloved child starves herself to death. I don't know what it's like to lose years to a sibling whose protest leaves no room for anything else. I don't know how it looks to those outside the family, uncomprehending, critical: 'Why don't you do something? Why don't you just *make* her eat?'

My eating disorder was a black hole that swallowed the whole family. My siblings were sidelined. My parents became haggard and embattled. They too were being watched and tried. We were public property; people whispered about us, judged us:

'It must be her parents' fault.'
'They should have spotted it sooner.'
'They put her under too much pressure.'
'I'll bet they told her to go on a diet.'

Mum told only one colleague. My sister told no-one. What could they say? It was distasteful, even obscene. I'd brought a plague upon our house. A sickness that infected everything – our lives, our jobs, our friendships. We knew no-one else in the same situation, and we had little support. It was just us, battling against the world. Just us, battling against one another.

At the young people's unit, counsellors probed me with questions:

'Has anyone ever touched you?'

No.

'Have you ever been physically abused?'

No.

'Is there something about your family you need to keep a secret?'

No.

They poked and prodded till my brain throbbed like an enormous bruise.

Getting nowhere, the team suggested family therapy, but, to protect my siblings, my parents refused. Ruth and Michael had suffered enough. So we sat stiffly together in a tiny, airless room. Mum, Dad, the counsellor and me. Oh – and a team of psychologists behind a two-way mirror. Very cosy.

Like many anorexics, I was a therapist's nightmare. I could have written textbooks on food, nutrition and the body. I didn't want to be there and I didn't 'need help'. Besides which, I didn't trust them. How could I? They were stripping away the only thing I had left.

We went round and round in circles. My parents, despairing and defensive. Me, alternately furious and mute. It felt like a prison line-up, with everyone a suspect. Everything was noted down, but no conclusions were reached. Instead, my slim file grew as fast as my waistline. It was assumed that, if I put the weight back on, every-thing would be fine. So that's what I did.

The promise

In a world of adults, I was fighting a losing battle. In spite of all my protests, the weight went on. I felt like a prize heifer, fattened for market and destined for slaughter. As the bones receded, I ricocheted between hope and despair. Externally, it seemed to be a fresh start. But from the inside, nothing had changed.

That's when I made myself a solemn vow. Whatever people wanted from me, that's what I would give them. If they asked me to jump, I would jump. If I had to put on weight, so be it. But they would never see the real me, or know what I was feeling. I would seal myself off, from people and from pain. I would give a performance, but never my heart.

On the outside, things were improving. I was a healthier weight and beginning to look like my old self. On the inside, the old drives remained. They just came out in new ways. I threw myself back into study with a vengeance. I worried constantly, about everything. The world seemed violent and unpredictable. Without the familiar outlets of exercise and food restriction, I needed new rituals to make it safe.

A new master

As my weight increased, so did my anxiety. But instead of 'fat', I found a new fear: germs. I became obsessed with contamination and cleanliness, scouring the *Reader's Digest* for articles on disease prevention. Anorexia had been usurped by another tyrant, just as dictatorial. It made little sense, but I felt powerless to stop.

At first I tried to avoid 'unsafe' areas. Public toilets, doctors' surgeries. But the contagion spread. 'Unsafe' quickly escalated to door handles or anything that someone else had touched. Instead of hiding food, I now stockpiled bars of soap, bought surreptitiously when Mum was distracted, or stolen from the school toilets. Pollution and dirt lurked on every surface. When I touched something unclean, I would feel unbearable levels of stress, a thick choking layer of panic.

The only solution was to scrub myself clean. I washed my hands and body obsessively, over and over, in a very specific order. The whole process took hours. Fingers, nails, wrists, arms – until the water ran red. Just one deviation invalidated my efforts, and I would have to start again. Yet the moment I finished, I'd touch something else and the process would begin afresh. It was madness, but I had to obey. If I didn't, something terrible would happen to me or the people I loved.

We returned to the centre, where they handed us more leaflets, illustrated with cartoons of happy families. After reading them through, we were none the wiser. According to the blurb, I now had 'obsessive–compulsive disorder' or 'OCD' (a common issue for recovering anorexics). Dad made a joke about Lady Macbeth, but no-one laughed. Instead, Mum shot him a murderous look and went to put the kettle on.

New laws

We added a new set of rules to the existing regime. In addition to the food diary and meal plans, there were now strict limits on my washing. Five minutes in the shower, and then someone would intervene. But the restrictions were impossible to police. At their worst, my hands had to be bandaged. The skin split open where I'd washed in neat bleach, with sores weeping blood. My siblings looked at me in disbelief, and I couldn't blame them. Cleaning products were locked away along with the scales. I felt trapped – in my own crazy head. Every day my world shrank further. But my anxiety was so terrible, I'd do anything to stop it.

Bit by bit, my weight and washing came under control. I had little choice. Everything I did was censored. But the old drives and self-hatred endured, undiminished. In fact, they grew worse. Yes, I'd channelled them into more 'appropriate' behaviours – academia, sleep – but I'd proved to myself and everyone else that I really was a freak. If this was recovery, it was only skin-deep.

A spiritual problem

For the sufferer, their eating disorder is an ally, their very best friend. It simplifies life and reduces it to a very simple equation. Stressed about exams, your body, your parents, life, death and the cosmos? No need. All that really matters is losing weight. It's the one universe over which you can proclaim, 'This is *mine*.' As the Minnesota study demonstrates, what's going on is never less than physical. But it's so, so much more. It's emotional, mental and, most importantly, it's spiritual. Unless recovery addresses these heart issues, it's just behaviour modification. More than this, it can exacerbate the flawed thinking that lies at the core.

What do I mean by a 'spiritual' problem? Well, like any disorder, anorexia starts and ends with our hearts.

Sure, we can throw in factors like celebrity role models and media coverage. But it throws up bigger questions than whether or not our clothes fit. What it means to be human, for starters. What gives us identity and worth. Life and death and everything in-between. What we *worship*.

This might sound archaic, especially if you're not a churchgoer. But we're all worshippers. The question is not *if* we worship; it's *what*. This could be anything – from work to relationships, from popularity to achievement. But something drives us. Something fills our dreams. And something gives our lives meaning. As my eating disorder took hold, I was just as 'religious' as I'd always been. I was still trusting in God. The difference was that this god had a small, rather than a capital 'g'. And surprise, surprise, it was a god that looked just like me. The god of performance, hard work, externals and rituals. A god that gave nothing of itself, but demanded everything in return.

Like any religion, anorexia is built on a mountain of beliefs about what constitutes life and death, salvation and sin, shame and redemption.

According to the *Bible*, sin is rejection of Christ – a refusal to receive from a giving God. It affects us all, but is illustrated perfectly in the girl who refuses to eat. With the goddess *Anorexia*, sin is redefined – and it's not just caloric. Instead, it's about a lack of self-control, the shame that comes with wanting and needing too much.

In the Bible, there *is* a problem with uncleanness, with sin and shame. It's a problem common to us all. Our sin *is* our separation from the life-giving God. And it's not something we can atone for ourselves. It requires a Scapegoat, someone perfect who can take our mess and all that it deserves. That's the salvation that only Jesus Christ can offer.

For the anorexic, however, 'fat' is the unforgivable sin. 'Fat' separates me from my god too – in this case, from the person I want to be. It also needs to be removed. In this model, salvation means atoning *for* myself, *by* myself: bearing my punishment in my own body. As I seek to recreate myself, my body becomes the scapegoat. I hate it and identify all that's wrong in my world with this lump of flesh. Yet at the same time, I also worship it, ritualizing and relishing every aspect of my self-imposed atonement.

Through the rituals, I separate myself from my messy, sinful flesh with its overwhelming desires. I will punish my body while I concentrate on the *real me* – almighty willpower. With my secret knowledge of exercise and nutrition, I can soar above my own fallibility. I can split myself into two and rise anew, born again to a new kind of humanity.

And what about the community of faith?

In the Bible, worship takes place in the context of a wider body where we are free to be ourselves and speak the truth in love. With anorexia, the opposite is true. I retreat into myself and cut myself off from relationships. I hide and I lie. I turn my hatred against myself and against anyone who comes close.

At the centre of the Christian faith is Christ's body and blood, broken and poured out for us. In the Lord's Supper we are reminded that we cannot save ourselves. We are needy – hungry for the bread of life. But in Jesus we have found a self-giving God who invites us to his table and feeds us. 'This man welcomes sinners, and eats with them' is what they said in the Gospels (see Luke 15:2), and it's just as true today. As we come in our brokenness, we know that we are *not* worthy, but we are welcome nonetheless.

At the centre of the anorexic faith is another body, also broken. This body is solitary. It is mine. And it is punished by me and for me. This continual sacrifice is proof that I *am* worthy after all. I wear my rules and rituals proudly, for all to see.

The drive towards self-improvement is relentless. The weight and exercise goals are never enough. The OCD and other rituals serve as sacraments. These things feel like freedom. But they enslave me. Each day more demands are added to the list. Each day my body shrinks along with my world.

The gospel of anorexia isn't good news at all. It is a system of works, of slavery, self-salvation and self-destruction. It feels like heaven, but leads to hell. It is a religion, as powerful and addictive as any cult.

What kind of recovery?

As part of my treatment, I was encouraged to get better by making a list of reasons to recover. On the plus side, I was reminded that I'd have 'clearer skin', 'more energy' and might 'get a boyfriend'. Also, other people would worry less. These are positive incentives. But weigh them against the promises of starvation, and they're less than nothing. Anorexia, remember, is the obsession that gives your life meaning. It's a way of conquering death: transformation into an indestructible new humanity. I'm not suggesting that the NHS doesn't understand the disorder or that I've got the solution. But our health service lacks the resources to treat it as a physical problem, let alone a metaphysical one.

Fighting these things with a checklist is as effective as throwing a bucket of water at a volcano. Talking yourself out of an obsession doesn't work, unless there is something – or someone – bigger to take its place. Worse still, it can reinforce the performance-based thinking that started it all off.

Instead of dealing with the underlying issues behind anorexia, I was encouraged to focus on externals and appearances. Weight gain, appropriate washing, normalized eating.

Instead of challenging my need to work hard and earn approval, I was given a programme of incentives and self-improvements. *Gaining weight is good.* When you do it, *you are good* – and you get to go out with your friends. *Losing weight is bad.* When you do it, *you are bad* – and you're grounded until further notice.

Just as I was shamed into God's kingdom, I was shamed into 'recovery'. Therapy involved looking for the answer 'within'. This sounds good, right? But what if, when you look inside, there's nothing there? Worse still, what if what's there is really rotten? What do you do with that? And where do you go when the experts can't help?

From the outside, it looked like recovery. I was a good girl again. I worked hard and even won a place at a top university. In the glossy magazines, this is where the story would end. But my so-called recovery sowed the seeds for a relapse, ten years later.

5 Recovery?

When is an anorexic 'recovered'? When they've regained weight? When mealtimes return to 'normal'? When they've kicked their exercise addiction? If that's the definition of recovery, then, aged eighteen, I had recovered. Looking back, however, I'm not so sure. These elements are part of the process – sometimes as essential first steps. But if the problem is seen as simply external, then the solution will also be skin-deep. Perhaps the *way* in which we 'recover' is as important as the fact that we do.

Paint job versus rebuilding

One of my guilty pleasures is trashy television. Top of the list are home-improvement programmes. The characters and locations may change, but the key ingredients are usually the same. First, the 'family in distress'. Surrounded by poor drainage, crumbling walls and lime-green lino, they've been trying to sell their home for years – with little success. In desperation, they call in the experts – a crazy interior designer and his merry band of builders. Depending on the production budget, they're then offered one of two options.

Option one is the quick fix. The requirements are minimal – twenty man-hours (give or take tea breaks), £50 cash and a pumping soundtrack. It's *Grand Designs* meets *The A-Team*. As the music starts, the SWAT team descends. Walls are painted, new curtains are hung, and a screen is nailed over the damp patches. No time to look at any structural problems, but not to worry: a few hanging baskets will disguise those cracks nicely. Fast-forward a few hours – and *voilà*! From a distance, the house seems transformed. Just don't peer too closely. Pray it doesn't rain. And whatever happens, don't come back in six months' time. If you do, you'll find nothing but a heap of rubble where your dream house once stood.

Option two is costlier and more difficult: a complete renovation, both inside and out. Success is not guaranteed, and it may take a lifetime. It's messy and frustrating. However, the end result is a building that's been genuinely transformed.

The 'recovery' process is not unlike these home-improvement programmes. You're working with people, not buildings, but the principles are just the same. You need a team of helpers who are committed to change. The question is: how much? Will it be a personal paint job – or a complete and costly overhaul?

Real change means exhuming the anxieties you've spent a lifetime burying. It's rebuilding the foundations, not just papering over the cracks. It's letting others in and admitting to weakness. Not just shifting the furniture, but lifting up the floorboards too.

Real change is bigger than body mass. It's deeper than replacing starving with stuffing. You might wash your hands instead of purging. You might place your hopes in exams instead of exercise. But, if this is all you do, then you're still a slave. You're still at the mercy of circumstance. Your desires may be sublimated, but they're nowhere near satisfied.

You can probably guess which of the recovery options I followed. Option one: the paint job. Don't get me wrong: in the short term, it saved my life. But long term, it simply deferred the battle.

Making it better

My 'quick-fix' recovery only confirmed the fears that had triggered my anorexia. It taught me this: my identity *did* depend on my weight. I *was* disgusting, and my mess *was* too much for others to handle. If I wanted to fit in, I had to bury my feelings. I *had* to perform.

No-one said this, of course. The accusations were real – but they came from inside my own head. I felt I owed an irredeemable debt: to my family, and to God. But, even if I'd donated both kidneys to medical research and plugged the hole in the ozone layer, it wouldn't have been enough. I couldn't atone for all the damage I'd caused.

I felt most guilty about hurting my family. Somehow, we'd survived an unthinkable horror – but only just. None of us were who we thought we were. None of us knew how to make it better. We acted as though nothing had happened and life could resume. But we couldn't go back and we couldn't forget. Anorexia was a dark monster that had cast its shadow across every room. It would not be dismissed. Though no-one spoke of it, when the conversation fell silent we could still hear it breathing.

My eating disorder had promised to eliminate the bad stuff: the feelings that I couldn't handle. Fear. Neediness. Lack of control. Ironically, however, it proved them instead. As my weight dropped, people really *were* staring at me in horror. As I exercised and starved in secret, I had a genuine reason to feel ashamed. I felt disgusting – and I looked disgusting too.

I couldn't turn back the clock. But rather than recognize my limits, I redoubled my efforts instead. Despair was impossible to live with, and I didn't want grace. I had to make it right. Slowly and reluctantly, I gained weight. I stopped hand-washing. I said the right things and found a new outlet for self-improvement: my old friend, academia.

This strategy worked – at least to begin with. I studied hard and won a place at Oxford University to study English literature. Everyone said how well I'd done, and I bathed in their approval. Finally – an end to the therapy and the weigh-ins and the whole sorry mess.

Before I left, my counsellor asked if I was planning to write about my experiences. 'Over my dead body,' I spat back. Anorexia was my deepest shame, the 'me' I wanted to leave behind. Writing was my future – the one thing I could be proud of. The past and the future would never, ever meet. Those years of madness and sickness were a temporary blip. Now my brains would be my salvation: now, I could vindicate myself.

But it didn't turn out quite as I had planned.

New world

Oxford was a little different from Belfast. Magical, but terrifying too. Our tutors wore tweed. We drank sherry and mingled in the masters' common room. During interviews, the girl beside me announced that she was a white witch. Choking, I stole a look at the other candidates. None of them appeared surprised: on the contrary, they radiated confidence and experience. Beside them, I felt like a little moth surrounded by emperor butterflies. But emboldened by the sherry, I took a deep breath and strapped on my cardboard wings. How hard could it be?

My college had a reputation for being intellectual, radical and left-wing. This, however, had passed me by. I'd 'picked' it because, in the prospectus, it was alphabetically first. The unofficial motto – 'Effortlessly superior' – was also at odds with my personal mantra: 'Try hard and don't get above your station.' I felt like a country mouse, chewing straw in the Big Smoke and gawking at the sights. But there was no time to take stock. People spoke with authority on topics I had never even considered. What, they asked, were my Views? I had no idea. I couldn't pronounce Nietzsche, let alone discuss him. As for New Labour? Er – refresh my memory on the old one. Plus, what on earth was a 'gap year'?

Oxford is designed for independent, self-motivated thinkers who question authority. As you've probably gathered, this is not me. Authority is my friend. I like rules, deadlines, targets, right answers, score cards and league tables. Without them, I feel anxious and a little lost. But these old certainties were way out of date. We were encouraged to question everything and to reread the classic texts through revolutionary lenses – Marxism, postmodernism and feminism. It was quite a shock. For years I'd fancied Mr Rochester, but it turned out he was secretly oppressing me. I felt as if I'd floated across the Irish Sea on a potato.

There were seven English students in my year, and the university operated a tutorial system. Yet while the class size was small, the demands were much greater. I was no longer the brightest in my year, and I was convinced that the college had made a mistake. Just thinking about essays filled me with panic. I spent days under my duvet, unable to face the thought of failure. Somehow, I got through. But it wasn't the introduction I had planned.

Being smart was the only thing that gave me value: without it I felt like a mollusc, de-shelled and set adrift. Blagging your way through a book you haven't read is tricky enough, but it's downright impossible when your tutor's a world authority on the subject. So much for 'redeeming myself with my brain'. It was time to find a new rock. But which one?

In the past, I'd moulded my body like a potter shaping clay. However, the results were not for public viewing: they were private, concealed beneath fabric and the posture of defence. I'd grown to tolerate how I looked, but it was a case of limiting the damage, rather than celebrating anything good. Now, however, the boundaries had shifted. From being clever but undeniably plain, I was now considered of average intelligence but (somehow) attractive. My impenetrable Irish burr was deemed exotic. My skin, so wan it glowed, was rechristened 'pale' and 'alluring'. In my second year I came second in the 'college babe' competition. I suspected people were laughing behind my back – but it wasn't a joke.

New weapons

The girls' school environment was gone too. In its place was a common room, sticky with testosterone and innuendo. All the boys seemed really friendly. But even gender was no longer fixed. Girls slept with girls. Guys wore 'guyliner' and even lipstick. In this new context, my body also meant something new. While it had once been a liability, now it became a tool. Deployed correctly, it was a weapon that could make even the smart guys act stupid. And so, armed with curling tongs and thick mascara, I decided to go on the attack.

'Fathers,' I cackled, 'lock up your sons . . . '

Yet though it might have seemed flattering, this new-found approval changed nothing: after all, it wasn't about me. My body was just a commodity, worth nothing in one environment, then valued in another. As brain stocks plummeted, I had simply shifted investments. Whether with studies or stilettos, I determined to gain acceptance, whatever it took.

New lifestyle

Compared to Belfast, university was Babylon. Everyone smoked and drank. Some took drugs. The other students were not just smarter than me, but comfortable in their own skin. It was astounding: boundless confidence oozed from every pore. They saw the world in a completely different light. In it *I* was foreign. *I* had an accent. *I* was different.

Even when subtitled, I was misunderstood. I warned friends darkly that oral sex would get them pregnant

– and was baffled when they laughed. People took me seriously when I was joking – and vice versa. Their sincerity was equally bewildering. They said nice things and didn't book-end them with retractions or jibes. For me, sarcasm was a way of life. Here, it was just plain rude.

In the midst of such upheaval, I became very depressed. My parents – endlessly patient – encouraged me to keep going. My sister wrote to me, and my brother told me jokes. Every night I cried down the phone. Every morning I swore I was going home. When I did go back for visits, I had to be peeled from my bedroom and pushed on to the plane.

'One more week,' my family said. 'Just give it a little longer.'

Miraculously, as the weeks grew into months, I started to feel less overwhelmed. Along with my family, my tutor, Sandie, provided endless tea and support. I made friends. And I discovered some exciting new pursuits: alcohol and cigarettes. For the good girl, this was a revelation – a way of switching off my worries and feeling in 'control'.

Something else changed. I fell in love. He was good-looking, popular, funny, confident and smart. All that I'd hoped for – except not a Christian. My beliefs were common knowledge: at college I had gained a reputation as the last virgin in Britain. 'No sex,' I said. 'Not until I'm married.' This was easy in theory. But the *Facts of Life* book had not prepared me for an actual relationship.

The results were predictable, but painful. We fought over my body like a piece of disputed territory, sometimes both on the same side. Every morning I vowed that we would sleep in separate beds. Every evening my limbs and willpower melted away. Eventually we settled on a compromise that made us equally unhappy. Our relationship was a source of pleasure and guilt, but I loved him and he loved me. Surely nothing else mattered?

As my social life caught fire, my spiritual ardour cooled. I felt too guilty to pray, and my Bible stayed shut. Occasionally I would visit the Christian Union but, without a beard and sandals, I imagined myself as a rebel. In reality, I was as edgy as my dad's golf jumper, but I forged ahead regardless. Church and Bible study didn't fit. I loved how alcohol made me feel – giddy and *light*, liberated from the constraints of everyday life. Getting drunk and dating a non-Christian were theoretically bad – but they also felt good. At church I'd been taught to put Jesus first and keep my body 'special'. But that body felt like an alien appendage: weird and ugly and different. Instead, I wanted someone who was physically there, to tell me I was beautiful and precious and worthwhile. I refused to give up my relationship or my freedom – not even for God.

I still believed in God, but it seemed unlikely he could have any faith left in me. Surely you went to him *after* you'd cleaned yourself up? In any case, I was probably beyond redemption. If Christianity was all about good behaviour, then I was heading straight for hell.

Nor did I know any Christians who could advise me. Well, with one exception. I had an Australian flatmate called Glen. Like me, he said he was a Christian. Like me, it was difficult to tell. We weren't in the same friendship group, and when we did collide, it was with the jolt of shame and mutual recognition. Once or twice we made it to church – but apart from this, we had little in common. Or maybe the opposite was true – perhaps we shared too much. In any case, he made me feel very uncomfortable. I told his girlfriend that she could do much better – and I meant it too.

* * *

Life continued. Astonishingly, I graduated with a degree in English literature. But what would I *do* with it? Writing was my passion, but this felt painful too. It was risky to pursue something I wanted so much – better not to try, than live with the inevitable failure. Instead, I moved to London and took a job with a public relations agency. For a short period I lived with my boyfriend and his family, but after four years we finally broke up. I was devastated. It hadn't been working, but without him I felt utterly lost. Friends rallied round and we hit the town. I drank more and ate less. Inside, however, I was full of questions: Did I really need another boyfriend? Or was I hungering for something else? The Lord had been my first real love, but we'd lost contact. Even if I'd dialled heaven, he would probably have ignored my call. So I stayed as I was: drinking, dancing and dating.

6 Religious

One afternoon while I was waiting for a train, something odd happened. A young woman approached me and asked if I wanted to join a Bible study. This seemed like divine intervention, so I readily agreed, and we arranged to meet the very next day.

It was the first in a series of increasingly intense studies. I was familiar with the Bible, but services at this church were nothing like the ones I'd attended back home. The main meetings took place in an old school. They lasted for hours at a time, with lots and lots of singing. Unlike some of the Christians I'd known, the people there were passionate and excited about their faith. They met almost every night, including weekends. They were totally committed to serving Jesus and used phrases like 'on fire' and 'sold out for God'. Many of them had given up their homes and jobs to serve the church – in fact, this was seen as completely normal. Most of them were young, good-looking and successful. More than this, they were overwhelmingly *friendly*. Everyone wanted to meet me. Everyone wanted to know my name. When was I getting baptized, they asked. Why didn't I leave my flat and move in with them?

This came as music to my itching ears. At last I'd found people who took religion seriously, real leaders who exhorted us to make converts and live better lives. Brains and beauty had made no difference to my life. It was time to Get Moral instead. I was even assigned my own 'discipler', to tell me how to use my time and money. This might have been overwhelming, but everyone was so nice. They made me feel really good about myself. When we were singing together with the candles and the music and the hugs, I finally felt that God might accept me. All I had to do was keep his commands. It made sense – to be forgiven the past, I had to work off my debts. Plus, rules were reassuring – you kept them or you didn't, and you knew exactly where you stood.

At the back of my mind, however, there lurked a few, niggling doubts. Something here didn't quite add up. It didn't fit with what I'd been taught in Sunday school. At the new church, they said they were following the original biblical model. But, in practice, we only studied certain books. James, for example: 'Do not merely listen to the word . . . Do what it says' (1:22). Or the Sermon on the Mount. Passages about giving, obedience and church authority. But nothing about God's forgiveness and unconditional love.

Questioning was discouraged and seen as evidence of a weak faith. Disagreement meant that you were immature, or worse: that you had a divisive spirit. If you didn't repent, your discipler would take you aside and haul you up before the leadership team or even the church. The safest strategy was to keep quiet and agree.

At first, I kept my anxieties to myself. They were a sign of my weakness, the work of the devil, trying to enslave me all over again. I channelled my doubts into better behaviour. I resolved to give up alcohol and stop going out – except for mandatory prayer meetings. Friends and flatmates voiced their concerns, but when I staggered home after church, I was too tired to talk. In any case, I'd been warned not to trust their advice. What had I been told? That this was the one true church. Those outside of it were deceived.

Everything began speeding up. I was told to leave behind my old friends and to move in with my discipler. Most importantly, I needed to get baptized. I'd been baptized as a child, but my old one didn't count. Without *their* baptism, they told me, I was going to hell. I wasn't so sure. Surely Jesus, and not some special water, brought you to God? Baptism was a *sign* that you trusted God – not salvation itself.

I thought it over and prayed it through. I was prepared to concede on every other issue, but not on this. The leadership team shouted and pleaded with me to repent. I was wilful, disobedient, deluded. Were they right? I dug in my heels. I had no-one to talk to, but in desperation I remembered Glen, my flatmate at university. He had moved back to Australia, but I'd heard that he'd 'found his faith' again in a major way. Desperate for help, I sent him an email. What did he think?

Glen responded immediately. Pretty soon he mentioned the word 'cult'. This seemed somewhat extreme, but I couldn't dismiss his opinion either. Something had happened to him in Australia, and he spoke with conviction of a life-changing relationship with Jesus. He knew his Bible and said it was about grace, not rules – Christ's work for us, not our work for him. Best of all, he was moving to London to work in a church close to my office. If anyone could help me, surely it was him.

Days after his arrival, Glen and I met my discipler to tell her I was leaving. There were tears and threats. But Glen refused to budge. Quoting Scripture, he fought my corner and led me out of the café and out of the church. He helped me to change my phone number and kept me going when my church friends cut me off.

'God will not forgive you for this betrayal,' they said.

'Nonsense,' said Glen (though in more colourful language). If God was who they claimed he was, no-one would be good enough for him anyway.

New church

The experience left me shaken, and it was some time before I could be persuaded to visit another church. But Glen got me along to his one: All Souls, Langham Place. For months I hid at the back and fled from contact. Yet gradually, I began to feel safe. The teaching there was simple and it made sense. We were encouraged to ask questions and to measure everything the ministers said against the Bible. They didn't ask for my money or tell me to give up my job. They spoke instead about the cross – the heart of Christianity. Jesus had to die for us – which meant that our problems were more serious than we realized. But Jesus *wanted* to die for us – which meant God's love was also greater than we could imagine.

This was so much more than I had hoped for. I had tried to clean myself up and I'd tried to rescue myself. But my efforts had only made things worse. They'd exposed a heart that was darker, more demanding and more deceitful than even I had suspected. A heart I couldn't understand, let alone change.

But perhaps someone else did – and could?

If the gospel was true, then it meant one thing: Jesus saw me and loved me – whatever I'd done and whatever I did. He wasn't waiting for me to fix myself. He didn't want me to earn my way. He wasn't fooled by my masks or my strategies. He gave himself to me, even in the midst of my mess. I started to pray. 'If you're there, God, show me it's true. Show me *you're* real.'

And amazingly, he did. The more I read about Jesus, the more persuasive and attractive he became. He wasn't who I thought he was: a well-meaning teacher or a guru. If all I needed were some helpful maxims for living, I could buy a magazine. Over and over again, Jesus had said he was God's Son. There was no room for misunderstanding. If he wasn't who he claimed to be, then he was a liar and a fraud.

In the church I'd just left, the Bible was a rule book, used to beat us into submission. At All Souls, it was the place where we encountered Jesus. Meeting him fired my heart. My old pastimes – drinking and partying – didn't give me the same buzz as before. Even my job seemed pointless and dull. So I made a decision. I handed in my resignation, told my flatmates I was moving out and applied to work as a lay assistant at All Souls. The job spec was caretaking with Bible teaching on top – dusting and doctrine, with the pay to match. But I was certain it was the right choice. I loved learning more about Jesus. It was wonderful to be part of such a caring and supportive staff and to read more of the Bible. For the first time, I felt like I was really living.

New job, old habits

Things were starting to make sense – yet old habits die hard. My new job was a fresh opportunity to work hard and earn respect. So that's exactly what I did: I volunteered for extra tasks, studied hard and prepared what I hoped were groundbreaking Bible studies.

In many ways, the Lord blessed these efforts. I met some amazing people and was able to encourage and care for others. I learned how to write talks and to share what I believed. Life felt exciting and hopeful once more. Yet the old drives were also beginning to resurface. While I was happy to keep God updated on my plans, I didn't want him to shape them. What I'd always suspected was being confirmed: I wasn't really a model, a thinker or a rebel. I was a 'good girl'. Here was an identity in which I could really invest. One that was perfectly suited to a religious environment.

Not everyone approved of this strategy. Glen, for starters: 'You do realize, don't you, that you can't do anything to earn God's approval? He *already* loves you.'

'Yes, yes,' I'd say.

Dear, simple Glen. My opinion of him had soared since university. He was one of the few people with whom I had always been myself – perhaps because, initially, his opinion seemed irrelevant. A lot had changed, and he might even have become my best friend – at least, until the government intervened. As I received confirmation of my new job, Glen too received a letter – from the Home Office: 'Dear Sir, your visa has expired. Please leave the country or go to prison.' A few days later, he was on a flight back to Australia.

Without Glen, I felt lonely and lost. We scoffed at suggestions of romance, but nonetheless spent every waking moment attached to a computer or a telephone. After months of sleepless nights (and eye-watering phone bills), I awoke to an email suggesting we were more than just friends.

'I think I love you,' he wrote. 'What do you reckon?'

For thirty-six hours I pondered my response. Finally, I replied. 'You know,' I typed, 'you might just be on to something.'

Over the next nine months that 'something' became a lot more concrete. Empowered by prayer and red wine (just for the take-off), I faced my fear of flying and went to meet Glen's family. They survived. He returned the favour by coming to Belfast to meet mine. Incredibly, he too survived. A few months later, on the steps of Sydney Opera House, he asked me to become his wife. This time I didn't hesitate and – between giggles – threw my arms around his neck.

And so, aged twenty-five, we were married. It was a brilliant day. The photos show two giddy youngsters, emboldened with the confidence of naivety, youth and (cheap) champagne. In the run-up to the wedding, I had lost a bit of weight, but we put it down to wedding nerves. After all, what bride-to-be doesn't slim down?

Glen was now working as a 'teaching pastor' at a church in central London. I was doing some PR for All Souls, but it was a new position and, despite my bravado, I felt inadequate and overwhelmed. I wanted to prove myself, but was paralysed by my own expectations. While it was kind of them to keep me on for as long as they did, I was unsuited to the role. My future – whatever it held – was not in marketing. It was time to find a new career.

Returning from honeymoon, I struggled to pick up the pieces of my old life. I had no job and, so I concluded, no purpose either. I became very depressed. As I rewound the events of my life, old wounds started to reopen. As a teenager, I'd almost broken up my family with my starving and scrubbing. At college I had been lonely and depressed. I was a terrible Christian who joined a cult. Finally, I had lost my job. It was a reminder of the labels I'd tried so hard to leave behind: 'Weird'; 'Unacceptable'; 'Lazy'. My résumé was useless, and so was I.

As my hopes subsided, I lapsed into old patterns. Food. Exercise. Busyness. Alcohol. I bought a fitness DVD and pounded a hole in the living-room carpet. I baked, dusted and cleaned the house, until every surface shone. I applied for jobs that were completely unsuitable, took them and then quit. Every day I felt more useless and ashamed. I wasn't bright or pretty or good. I was a big, fat, ugly mess.

Yet, even in these disappointments, there were a few chinks of light. I'd been volunteering at the church where Glen worked, and my old boss recommended me to the vicar there. I discovered that I was good at working with kids – perhaps because we think in similar ways. I could explain things in a way they understood. I identified with their intensity, the way they related to the world, their curiosity and hunger to learn. So when the church offered me a full-time position as children's worker, I leapt at it. I wasn't completely useless after all! Here was my chance to prove it.

It seemed that Glen and I were finally back on track – ministry dynamos, high on gifting, if not maturity. We applied to study together at Bible college. To help fund my studies, we agreed that I would keep doing children's work, but cut back on other commitments. Glen wanted me to study part-time and work part-time, but I refused to listen. Instead, I insisted that I would study full-time and work as well. The hours didn't add up, but that was irrelevant. Having failed in every other area, I was determined to prove my worth. I wasn't a crazy thirteen-year-old, destroying her family. I wasn't a depressed student, unable to get out of bed. I wasn't a drunken sell-out or a deluded cult member. I wasn't just a wife, dependent on her man. From the wreckage of the past, I would emerge transformed and radiant. I would build myself a future – and with it, a brand-new name.

7 Relapse

One of my favourite poems is called: 'Not Waving but Drowning'.[3] The title says it all. You can appear to the world like you've got it together – right place, right time, right behaviour – yet still be in serious trouble.

From the outside, I looked like a great Christian. Glossy, high-functioning and motivated. An all-singing, all-dancing children's worker, student and super-achiever. Not all of this was bad. I worked hard. I loved Jesus, and I loved the kids in my care. The church was a fantastic training ground and taught me a lot. Nonetheless, at the heart of a thriving ministry beat a commitment to proving myself. I appeared to be waving. I was drowning instead.

Idols, you see, are not always easy to spot. They are subtle and adaptable. Given the right packaging, they'll flourish as readily in churches as in temples. And, in my experience at least, they rarely present themselves as enormous, gilded cows.

As a children's leader, Bible student and trainee minister's wife, I knew all the right answers. At Bible college I submitted textbook essays on 'the gospel'. I even spoke about it at church. But the truths I taught to others were like the sandwiches I fed my husband. Not for me. Other people needed grace. *My* problems required a more sophisticated approach.

The ultimate makeover

My life had, once again, become a series of overwhelming demands. Lectures, assessments, church work, *marriage*. I felt like a child – overwhelmed and out of control. But I needed to stay busy, and I was too proud to ask for help. As the old feelings resurfaced, so did the old solutions. I craved another makeover. But with what? Moral performance? Academia? Looks? In a stroke of genius, I resolved to pursue all three. Good girl, smart girl, pretty girl. Just watch me go.

The product

First up for vindication was my brain. I'd messed up university first time around, so this was an opportunity to make it right. Yet Bible college was not like Oxford. For starters, I was a woman at a male-dominated institution. I was also a children's worker. Would I be taken seriously? I resolved to prove my worth among the big boys and carve out a role beyond 'Glen's wife'. But it was harder than I imagined. For many students, this was a second or third degree, and standards were high. Others had made huge sacrifices to be there: academic, personal and financial. We wanted to make the time count. Yet, while most were inspired by God, my motivation was a great deal more selfish. No matter. I kept my head down, avoided the wives' groups and focused on what was really important: my grades.

Once more I started getting up early. Scribbling through lunch. Cramming over dinner. Over and over, I rewrote my papers – furious arguments in which I peppered imaginary opponents with doctrinal bullets.

Time wore on and my obsession grew. My brain was like a scythe, glittering and sharp, slashing and destroying all adversaries. I experienced flashes of tantalizing clarity, where I felt that I was on the edge of a great discovery. In everything I saw answers – codes and systems, keys to unlock the universe. Every tick from my tutors was a vindication – a fist in the face for the voices telling me I was nothing.

It wasn't just study that preoccupied me. As I'd learned in the past, good grades were not enough. I wanted to look as powerful as I felt. Time for phase two of the makeover: a shiny new body to match the brain.

The packaging

As impoverished students, we couldn't afford new clothes, so I trawled charity shops instead. Much more than a hobby, it was a quest of deadly seriousness, demanding the same intensity and rigour as my studies.

I spent hours upon hours sifting through garments and hunting for 'the right look'. I amassed hundreds of costumes, suitable for every situation. One for every woman I had ever admired, from earth mother to head of state. One for every size – from zero to plus. Every role I'd played in the past. Every ambition I had for the future.

Career Emma, sharp-suited and heeled. The children's worker, an explosion of colour and neon stripes. The vicar's wife, a delicate froth of florals. Tie-dyes for the student. Lycra for the fitness fanatic. Tweed for the academic. 'Edgy Emma', the Londoner, zipped up in leather. For every fantasy, I had a garment. Scores of outfits but no-one to wear them. Like a rag doll, dreaming of Barbie, I didn't wear a single one. Not even once.

Just as academia offered solutions, so each new outfit promised redemption and renewal. In the bedroom, clothes spilled out of every wardrobe. Sartorial possibilities strode across my brain in an endless catwalk. But there they all stayed, bagged and unopened. On the hanger, they whispered salvation. But in practice, they were too good for me – at least for now. One day I would burst, triumphant, from this chrysalis. I had to believe that. I would put on my new clothes, and they would fit, and I would fit, and it would be wonderful. Not yet. But if I just worked harder. Collected a few more outfits. Wrote better essays.

Lost a little weight.

It was such a small beginning. I just wanted to get fit, that was all. A bit of exercise. First thing in the morning, before lectures began. Nothing wrong with that – right?

Running made me feel in control. It gave me a high. With every stride, I outstripped the spectre of the past and the fears of the present. I ran and I ran and I ran. From the frightened thirteen-year-old with no friends and no clue. From the twenty-five-year-old with no job and no hope. I ran until my legs ached, my lungs burned and I could no longer think.

Each day I pushed the boundaries of my endurance. I got up earlier. Exercised harder. I developed rituals and routines – for exercise, working and, most of all, for food. My portions shrank. I cut out fats. Carbs. Proteins. Lost some more weight.

Mentally and physically, I was pushing, pushing, pushing. I exercised. I shopped. I worked and I starved. A machine, not a person. Body and mind, toning, training, turning. I lost sense of time. Hours merged into days. Weeks became months. It tasted like freedom, but my world was contracting instead. I laughed when Glen suggested a holiday – there simply weren't enough hours in the day. Our marriage was not a priority: it could take care of itself.

Locked inside my head, I had no space for relationships – with my husband, with friends and, most of all, with God. Tutors spoke warmly of the 'living Lord', as did the other students. Yet the more I studied him, the further away he seemed – a collection of attributes, not a Person. In my head, I understood that God was 'good' and 'loving' and 'fair' – but I couldn't relate these things to my own experience. The truths of the Bible were drowned out by other, louder voices.

'You're nothing,' they said. 'You're not *enough*.'

Hunger

This hunger is something that I've always felt. Not just for food – but for everything: from money to recognition. 'More!' is the cry of my heart. 'Give me more.' The emptier

I feel, the more I need. I don't deserve it. But I want it, more than anything. I'm a human chasm, a vortex of insatiable longing. And I'll do whatever it takes to slake that thirst. Overworking. Overexercising. Overdrinking. Overspending. Overcleaning. There's just one problem. Whatever the fuel – clothes, booze, thinness – 'more' is never enough.

The word 'anorexia' means 'loss of appetite'. This is a stunning misnomer. Of *course* you're *hungry*. You might as well be an enormous pair of lips and teeth. Hunger is your pulse. It's what gets you out of bed. Hunger drives you forwards, when your body wants to give up. It's your first thought and, without help, it will be your last breath too. You're dominated by your appetites – for affirmation, acceptance and everything you want but can't quite get.

I've always had a fear of 'running out'. I used to laugh at my granny, queuing for credit at the grocer's and reusing tea bags till the water ran clear. Yet she lives on in the thirty-four-year-old who stockpiles toilet rolls and tinned tomatoes. I suspect this is part of what it means to be human: a shoring up against spiritual and material deficit, a defence against drought, death and disappointment. In myself, however, need is something I have always despised. It feels like weakness. It makes me vulnerable and exposed. I won't be dependent. I'll earn it. I'll crush those desires – or die trying.

Of course, there's another way to deal with hungers: denial. If you repress your longings then life becomes greyer, but simpler too. You're in charge of your weight and your life. Now, instead of those desires killing you, you're killing them. At least, that's how it feels.

From the outside, however, the situation looks very different – especially once the disorder has taken hold. By the end point, everyone can see you're in terrible danger. But initially at least, the descent is slow. Recriminations abound. 'Why didn't you stop her?' 'How did it get so bad?' But that's to mistake the nature of the problem. Anorexia isn't a sudden plunge into the abyss. Silent, stealthy and secretive, it's a gradual attrition of body, mind and soul.

History repeating

As I grew worse, the warning signs became harder to ignore. I'd been here before, and I knew the ending. Part of me said, 'Do it alone.' But I was conscious of another voice, one that spoke with authority. Not my husband's, not even mine. I heard him when I prayed. 'No,' God said, 'you can't.'

For once, I listened. I made an appointment to see my doctor.

Once in the surgery, I regretted my decision. How pathetic! What on earth was I doing? Burning with shame, I tried to explain.

'I've got a history of anorexia.' I cleared my throat. 'And I think . . . I think it's starting up again.'

The doctor examined me and then my records. She looked concerned.

'Your BMI is dropping very quickly,' she said. 'You can't afford to lose any more weight. I'm referring you to a specialist treatment centre – but I'll warn you now, the waiting lists are considerable. Let's see what they say, and we'll go from there.'

I nodded gamely, but inside I was panicking. Anorexia gave me an identity that I hated, but one I also sought. A sense of purpose. An exemption from the demands of life. A voice – demanding care and attention, while repulsing those who got too close.

Anorexia was my very best friend. She worked me hard, but she comforted me too. She'd accompanied me through most of the major rites of passage. She gave my life meaning, structure and value. When other people let me down, she was there. When I disgusted myself, she had the solution. Did I really want to give her up? I told myself, 'Yes.' But I felt her grip on me tighten.

A few months later, I received an appointment for the eating disorders' wing of a local hospital. In the meantime, I'd redoubled my efforts to lose weight, and, despite my protestations, people were beginning to notice.

'Are you OK?' they asked. 'You don't look well.'

I retreated further. 'I'm fine,' I said. 'I'm seeing a doctor.' Subtext: *Leave me alone. It's none of your business.*

Getting help for an adult with anorexia is very different from treating a minor. It's still an addiction. But unless the sufferer asks for support, there's a limit to what others can do. I was no longer under my parents' authority. There were no teachers to watch me at school, and no-one to force-feed me spaghetti. Glen tried his best, but to no avail. I refused to cede control.

We went to the hospital. The nurses there challenged me, but they were greatly overstretched. There were barely enough places for those who wanted help, let alone the ones who didn't. As I stood on the scales, I fingered the weights in my pockets. Yes, I was eating. No, I hadn't lost weight.

'Come back in a month's time,' they said, 'and we'll monitor your progress.'

'It's fine,' I repeated. 'Everything is fine.'

I jogged home and resolved to eat less. But there was nothing left on my plate to cut.

A month later and I was back. The wards were full of patients – skeletons, thinner than me, fighting the feeding tubes with every breath. In the waiting room I scanned magazines of models with bodies like mine. An elderly woman sat opposite me, shrivelled and bent. But when she spoke, it was with the voice of a child.

'My mum's coming to pick me up,' she told the woman at reception.

The buzzer rang and in came a woman in her forties. She led her daughter – the wizened old lady – outside. We watched in silence as they walked, slowly, to their car.

Another buzzer rang. Time for my weigh-in. I had a belly full of water and lips primed with lies, but there was no denying it: my weight had dropped. My ankles were swollen, and my body was now covered with a layer of fine fur. When I stood up, I felt dizzy, and climbing stairs was becoming impossible.

'If you keep going like this,' they said, 'you're going to collapse. We can put you on a waiting list for in-patient treatment, but you're not a priority just yet.'

It was almost funny: I couldn't afford to get worse. But to get treatment, I had to lose more weight.

The cost

There are many ways for an eating disorder to destroy you, not all of them obvious. First, there are the physical effects. Dehydration. Muscle atrophy. Paralysis. Gastrointestinal bleeding and ruptures. Chronic fatigue. Kidney failure, osteoporosis, arthritis. Cramps, bloating, incontinence, hair loss. Gum disease, insomnia, hyperactivity, infertility, seizures, heart attacks. I didn't realize it at the time, but my body had already suffered irreparable damage.

Of course, that's not all. There are psychological issues too. Loneliness. Waves of despair and sheer exhaustion. Paranoia. Fear. Isolation. Panic attacks. Depression. Shame. For every death that makes the news, there are thousands of hidden casualties. They may disintegrate a little more slowly, but they end the same way.

Then there are relationships. Impossible, of course. Perfection demands sacrifice. Family. Friends. A partner. Children. Forget them all. Intimacy is impossible without truth – and you're a walking lie. Furtive, guilty and defensive, you trust nothing and no-one. Those who try to reach you are swiftly repelled, blasted by a torrent of righteous anger, tears, hysteria and hostility: 'Why don't you trust me?'

'We do trust you. But not your anorexia.'

Neither of you say it, but you're thinking the same thing: *What's the difference?*

Not that it matters. Relationships are unthinkable. 'Ana' is all that you need. She's your mother, your lover, your sister, your friend. She's jealous, demanding, intoxicating and deadly. And above all else, she will not share.

Anorexia has a terrifying gravitational pull: it sucks in those in its orbit. Sufferers don't want to be lifted out – they want others to join them in the darkness. Within our marriage, I demanded Glen's companionship – but always on my terms. I clung to him, but spurned his advances. No lights. No noise. No sudden movements. I begged him not to leave me, but couldn't look him in the eyes. Both sets of parents lived overseas, and I warned him not to betray me to family or friends. Over time we forgot how our marriage had been: after all, every couple has their struggles. The madness became normalized – and we made room for our new housemate.

Help!

This is not to say we didn't seek help. As well as medical assistance, we searched in vain for psychological and spiritual aid. Glen contacted more than twenty counsellors on either side of the Atlantic, but only a few even wrote back. Again and again, we poured out our story, and it grew cheaper each time. We met Christians with years of pastoral training and experience who told us that my problems were just 'too big'. Others, baffled, shook their heads: there was nothing they could do. And there was no-one they could recommend either. Glancing at the qualifications lining their walls, we pleaded: 'What about *you*?' Sadly they weren't *that* qualified. The NHS, we were told, were the experts. Those experts said I wasn't sick enough for further treatment.

There were, however, a few lifelines in the storm. Normal Christians, untrained and unsure of what to do, but who prayed, kept praying and stood with us in our misery. Tutors. Classmates. Strangers whose kindness pierced a hole in the gloom. One, a counsellor called Dick, travelled hours to listen to our story. He didn't have a solution, but neither was he cowed by the scale of our problems. He pointed us back to a big God who could deal with our mess and to a community who genuinely cared. Even in our helplessness, Christians like him helped us to not give up.

New threats

While necessary, the prospect of community was also terrifying. Glen and I were approaching the end of our three years at college, and he would soon be ordained as a minister. For someone like me – wedded to order and routine – it was an appalling prospect.

Where would we live? Glen's job could take us any-where – from a sprawling rural vicarage to a cramped inner-city flat. Yet, by this point, I was struggling to leave the house. Strangers gawked at me, and I had panic attacks, chest pains and headaches that lasted for days at a time.

There was also the question of my role. A curate is a vicar with their 'L-plates' on, making me a 'curate's wife'. As a job description, it filled me with nausea. I was baffled by what a *woman* should be, let alone a superwoman. From a virtual hermit who spurned social contact, I would now be expected to share my husband and home with hundreds of strangers. My new calling was as the embodi-ment of godly womanhood – an all-feminine, all-fragrant dispenser of wisdom, hospitality and tray-bakes. Someone unlike me, in every way. It was unthinkable. I was too ashamed to meet my old friends, let alone make new ones. I had tried and tried and tried, and I couldn't, I just couldn't fail again.

But the voices wouldn't stop. In fact, they grew louder. A friend asked if I was dying – and we had no idea what to say.

'We're getting all the help we can.'

This was the truth. Exhausted, we had reached the end of our resources. No-one could help and nothing could be done. I stopped returning phone calls and messages.

'It's fine,' I muttered. 'I'm fine.'

Physically and mentally, however, I'd already checked out.

Retreat

From this point onwards, life left me behind. I'd start a hundred tasks and finish none. I wanted to go running, but couldn't walk up the stairs. I wanted to work, but couldn't remember what I was teaching. When people spoke, I watched their lips but I couldn't recognize the words. The lines on my textbooks melted one into the other. Finally, unwillingly, I dropped my modules at college. The last one to go was my long dissertation. Its subject? 'An Analysis of Eating Disorders'.

Trying to explain

Mapping this period is still very difficult. Some of my memories have sunk without a trace. There are echoes of conversations, but it's like watching a slow-motion film of someone else. Moth-eaten months that crumble to the touch.

Others, however, are luminous and urgent. These ones are like bodies in the water, resurfacing suddenly and without warning.

I can vividly remember lying in the Accident and Emergency department, hooked up to a heart monitor and trying to breathe. The first clumps of hair lying across the pillow. And Glen, carrying me up the stairs to our flat, when I could no longer walk.

'It's fine. I'm fine.'

I want to explain to you what it feels like to be slipping downwards. The constant exhaustion. Bitter cold – even in summer. The first chest pain. The panic attacks. The rituals and the rules. My pen trembles in my fingers, but the words are stuck.

I want to paint my husband – the bravest, most beautiful human I know. I want to show you him: loving me, caring for me, serving me, fighting for me. His desperation, bewilderment and despair. The people he contacted for help. The loneliness of marriage to a wife who won't be touched.

I want to explain what it feels like to live with an addict. A cold, implacable enemy masquerading as someone you love. A will of iron that, unbending, breaks those who try to resist it. The lies. The secrecy. The promises. The anger. The pleading. The grief.

Little by little, the person you know changes. She's furtive. She withdraws. She laughs at you when you question her. She closes down. She goes on the attack. She hides the evidence.

Her excuses are faultless:

She's already eaten.
She's meeting friends.
She's working late.
Don't you trust her?
Can't you see how hard she's trying?
She's a big girl.
She's just tired.
Everything's fine.
Stop being so *controlling*.

For those watching, there's only helplessness and horror.

You see, the face of anorexia is a terrible thing. It's not a glossy model in a perfume ad. Or a delicate patient, emaciated, yet beautiful. It's a cadaver, cloaked in sequins, modelling her new clothes. It's a starving animal, circling the empty cupboards. A creature, splattered in vomit, blank-eyed and vacant. A child, rocking back and forwards in the darkness. Foraging through the bins for mouldy bread. Chewing it and spitting it out. It's a face frozen in a rictus grin, mouthing lies. 'I'm fine,' it says. 'Everything is under control.'

I want to rip off its skin: to show you this, and so much more – but I can't find the words.

Maybe other anorexics look in the mirror and see a fat person. Maybe others pursue size-zero perfection. For me, this was never the goal. In some senses, I *wanted* to appear as hideous as I felt – to scream aloud what I could barely whisper. Greater still was the fear: fear of exposure and fear of losing control. But the more I tried to escape, the more I became what I most despised.

For centuries, Christian thinkers have spoken of our will as being 'bound'. They don't mean that we're robots and can't do what we want. It's a deeper imprisonment than this. The bondage of the will means that we *only* do what we want. We follow our desires all the way to the basement – and then we lock the door. *That's* our slavery.

This was my experience. I didn't set out to die. But I was drawn towards self-destruction. Every choice seemed to mire me deeper – no matter how I tried to wriggle free. I thought I could use anorexia as a way to live. In reality, it was using me – and its trajectory was death. Internally, it was 'what I wanted'. Externally, I was totally and demonstrably lost.

Addicts talk about 'rock bottom'. It's sometimes presented as the last great hope for those who can't be helped – a jolt from outside to set things straight. There is, however, one serious problem: you can't predict who will make it that far. Or if they'll ever get back up. No-one who dies of an eating disorder planned it that way. And I'm under no illusions: this could so easily have been me.

Many people have suffered organ failure or heart attacks at body weights that were higher than mine. What preserved me was the mercy of God. In the same way, only he could give me back a life. But this seemed beyond the realms of even divine possibility.

Like everything else, Glen's ordination passed in a blur. I smiled and waved, but couldn't digest an apple, let alone a conversation. College was over, and I'd discharged myself from the NHS programme. They had nothing more to offer us, and anyway we were moving out of London. Nothing mattered – not the church we would be going to in Eastbourne, not my family or friends, not my husband, not my studies, not my life. My body was shutting down, and with it my tenuous grasp on reality.

Ground Zero

I was tired. Bone-tired. Tired of living, tired of fighting, tired of trying to make sense of what was real and what was false. The past was a mess, and the future was formless and frightening. As for the present – all that existed was the hallway between my bedroom and the bathroom. The hallway in which I now lay.

Too weak to get back up.

Too broken ever to recover.

8 Revelation

There's no expert on recovery like the anorexic herself. Even as she strides towards destruction, she's convinced that everything is under control. As Glen and I moved from London to Eastbourne, this was how I felt. I had never been more enslaved. Yet I was never more certain of my own strength.

Self-help

Other people might die from anorexia, or sink without trace. *I* was different. The details were hazy, but I knew I could do it: I could turn my life around. Perhaps I'd wake up miraculously cured. Or drift naturally towards 'health' – without weight gain or effort, of course. One thing was certain: I didn't need help. Recovery was my affair, and mine alone. I would do it myself. No-one would force it upon me. No-one would tell me how to live.

Where did God fit in all this? For a Bible-college graduate, it's an obvious question. Yet, the way I saw it, God's business was spiritual and not physical. It's not just that I was running from the truth – I genuinely couldn't see it. I felt that, in most senses, I was living as he'd want. Spirituality had nothing to do with the day-to-day physicality of life. It was an escape from it, to a 'higher' realm.

God owned my soul, but my body was mine. If I kept going to church, praying and reading my Bible, then there was no real problem. I wasn't a brilliant Christian. But if I worked hard, I'd get there – wherever 'there' was.

Then I had a brainwave. I decided that I'd employ God in an advisory capacity – a bit like a consultant. Both of us were busy, so I'd make it simple. I would press the lever marked 'repentance', he would do his redemptive thing, and then we could both return to the business of real life. A temporary alliance, but with mutual benefits. He could take some of the credit, but I'd do my bit too; after all, I didn't need charity.

In my mind's eye I saw myself: modestly testifying to a packed and admiring stadium.

'It was a remarkable recovery,' I would demur. 'But I can't take *all* the glory. The Lord certainly helped.'

Events didn't work out quite as I'd planned. Not even close.

Arrivals and departures

We had been in Eastbourne for several months. Our new church was welcoming, but I rebuffed every advance. No-one knew how sick I was. My family had other worries too, right on their doorstep. Granny Black had been unwell for some time, and was becoming more and more confused. She stayed at home for as long as possible, but it became clear that she needed twenty-four-hour care. Mum said little on the phone, but her silence spoke volumes. Though I'd lost interest in everyone and everything else, I couldn't get Granny out of my head. So, on impulse, I booked a flight home to see her.

Mum picked me up at the airport. She looked grey, and her eyes were red. As she saw me, she flinched. We sat in the car together, like strangers.

'Emma,' she said, 'you look terrible.'

But I was no longer thirteen.

'I'm fine,' I insisted. 'I'm getting all the help I need.'

Next day I went to see my granny. Dad warned me: 'She might not recognize you, love. She's really sick.'

Sure enough, the woman in the bed looked like a ghost. She was a cut-out of her former self, shrunken and frail. Then again, so was I. I took her hand and searched her face. Would she know who I was?

Stroking her fingers, I thought of the adventures we'd shared. Drowsy afternoons spent watching old black-and-white films or sharing a jigsaw. Cresting traffic together atop the double-decker bus, and chasing pigeons from the swaying lines of washing. Wrestling over dominoes. Strawberry-picking in the blazing sun, the juice staining our teeth and running down our chins.

Sunday mornings at church, sinking into her soft bulk, and giggling as she jerked awake during the sermon: 'I was only resting my eyes.' Granny's generation didn't talk about such things, but she also knew Jesus – and it was another, unspoken link between us.

Best of all were the sick days from school, when I could keep her all to myself. Outside the rain beat down against the pavement. Indoors Granny made sense of life, holding it together with her hugs and homemade soup.

I looked at her, this woman whom I loved. And I saw that she was dying.

The words choked in my throat. 'Granny. I love you. I really, really love you.'

She turned her head and curled her fingers over mine. Then she looked at me, full in the face. In her eyes I saw wisdom and humour and recognition.

'Emma,' she said. 'Emma. I love you too.'

She knew my name. And for a moment, everything stopped.

Despite her sickness, Granny was there. And if she was, then maybe I was too.

As I boarded the plane, I felt dizzy and frightened. Nonetheless, something had stirred. Glen tried to hug me at the airport, but I wouldn't be touched. I felt almost nothing – bar the gentle imprint of my granny's fingers against mine.

Life returned to 'normal'. I promised my family I was getting better. Our new church tried to help, but my sickness sealed us off.

'Take as much time as you need,' they said. 'Have a holiday.'

Friends offered us their cottage by the Welsh coast. On impulse, we accepted and drove like fugitives pursued by the night. When we arrived, I went for a run along the beach. Glen sat in the kitchen and ate his sandwiches alone.

Next day we both slept late. When I awoke, my phone was flashing with a voicemail from Mum.

'Call me,' she said.

But I already knew. Granny had gone.

Dazed, Glen and I sat in the kitchen. We talked about going home for the funeral, but who were we kidding? I wasn't well enough to make the journey, and even strangers looked at me with pity and disgust. Instead of helping, my presence would have been a shocking distraction. I decided I would stay away.

It was an excruciating decision. But the pain was an awakening: like hunger, but not for food. I wanted to smell Granny's clothes and touch the things she had touched. To look with her eyes, one last time – and to see what she saw. To gather up her warm traces before time smoothed them away.

Most of all, I wanted to go home.

Something in me had broken. I wanted to be with people. People who could bridge this terrible loneliness. People who understood, who knew her. For the first time in months, I needed to speak. 'Granny.' That's what I wanted to say. *'Granny.'*

Without thinking, I picked up a pencil. It had been many years since I'd last tried to write. In the crucible of perfectionism, my words had melted away, leaving me frustrated and dumb. Up until now, I had had nothing to say.

My fingers felt awkward and rusty. But as I thought about Granny, they began to unfurl. Memories sprang, unconstrained, across the page. Her warmth. The way her eyes crinkled when she was trying not to laugh. Her appetite – for food and life and people. Her (selective) deafness. The steely insistence that, diabetes or no diabetes, she would definitely be having pudding. *With* cream.

Even through tears, she could still make me laugh.

I put down the pencil and picked up the phone. Though I couldn't be at the memorial service, there were words I needed to say. I called home and Mum picked up. For a moment, grief bridged us but, under the weight of my sickness, it buckled and broke. We stumbled towards speech before she passed me to Dad.

'If you can send us something in the next few hours,' he said, 'we'll read it out at the funeral.'

The house where we were staying was on the Welsh coast. It had no landline, let alone any Wi-Fi. From time to time, however, we could pick up a connection, usually just for a minute. As I switched on the computer, I prayed. 'Please, God, help me get this to my mum.'

A few moments later, the internet icon flickered, just long enough for me to email what I'd written. As soon as the document was sent, we lost the connection and it never returned.

I called home. 'Did you get it?'

'Yes,' said Mum. A pause. 'And you got her. In what you wrote – you got her, exactly right.'

The day of the funeral passed in a blur. I belonged with my family, but I'd made choices that barred me from their fellowship. What kind of creature had I become? I paced the hall in search of answers, but none came. Sleep too was impossible.

Game over

I sat in front of the fire, staring past the flames as they licked and spat in the grate. In trying to save myself, I had destroyed everything I had said I loved. I had come to the end of myself: I knew nothing.

In this extraordinary book Emma Scrivener opens a door into life with anorexia – she courageously allows us access into a desolate place with a very unwelcome visitor. Thank God for his saving grace and hope in Jesus Christ and for the fact that he has his grip on this precious woman telling her story. He will undoubtedly use these words for his purposes in the lives of others. Essential reading for any who are touched by the realities of anorexia.

Rachel Baughen, trustee of Keswick Ministries and UK Director, Kipepeo Designs

I could not put this book down. I have not read anything about eating disorders that approaches this book in clarity and insight. Beyond the weight loss lies a private world of perfectionism, shame and self-hate, which is not addressed by re-feeding and to which even those who are closest are denied access.

We are perhaps too quick to leave these kinds of bewildering problems to 'professionals'. This author is balanced about the value of medical intervention but also its limitations. She is very affirming of those who could bear to draw near and support, but is utterly clear that the route to deliverance and wholeness for her was in knowing the love of Jesus. *A New Name* she is light not just on anorexia, but on all kinds of self-harm and its effects on families. It is a very helpful book, heartening and enlightening.

Dr Annie Gemmill, GP

Emma Scrivener's reflections on her battle with anorexia are both a reality check and a road to recovery. She uncovers the roots of shame in her life, challenges controlling behaviours and chooses to receive the name that God offers her. Compelling and powerful reading which stays rooted and honest to the end.

Revd Will van der Hart, Director of Mind and Soul Foundation

Right from the start, I was gripped by this story. It is both frightening and fun, but most of all it gives hope when it seemed all was lost. Emma has fought back and, through her writing, will help many others, not only those with anorexia, but also those

who want to understand more fully why they act and behave in destructive ways.
Greta Randle, CEO Association of Christian Counsellors and author of Forgiving the Impossible? From Abuse to Freedom and Hope *(IVP)*

A moving and beautifully written book for all who want to think through what it is to be human. Utterly enthralling and eye-opening, it exposes just how very deep our problems go, and yet how healing is Christ. This is going to turn lives around.
Dr Michael Reeves, Head of Theology, UCCF

A New Name is a graphic account of a woman's slide into anorexia and her physical, emotional and spiritual struggle to break free. It gives insight into this complex condition and charts a way forward. Gritty and realistic, there is nothing triumphalist about this auto-biography. Read it to gain understanding and empathy.
Sheila Stephen, counsellor and supervisor; lecturer in women's studies, Wales Evangelical School of Theology

Beautifully written, shocking, searingly honest, inspiring. This book made me laugh and weep. I recommend it for those struggling with eating disorders and for those who try to support them. The most helpful description of anorexia I have ever read.
John Wyatt, Emeritus Professor of Neonatal Paediatrics at University College London, Chairman of the Christian Medical Fellowship Study Group, board member of Biocentre and of the London Institute for Contemporary Christianity

Emma has written a powerful book that provides a deeper insight into the mass of conflict that can precede an eating disorder, and the devastation of life that can ensue from it. She writes with vividness, passion and character, drawing upon the experience of her own fervent search for real answers. Sufferers, carers and clinicians alike will benefit from the information provided and the hope for recovery that is engendered.
Dr Ken Yeow, consultant psychiatrist in eating disorders, Belfast, Northern Ireland

Clothes and possessions hadn't worked. Academic achievements felt empty. Morality – my rules – seemed to offer redemption, but choked me instead. The rituals that promised salvation were iron-forged manacles that took me to hell.

I'd made my home in the darkness. I'd forgotten everything but myself. When the light came, I shrank from it, but, without God, I had no self to speak of.

This was it: the end. There was nowhere left to go.

In desperation, I cried out to the God I'd fought so hard to escape.

'Lord,' I said, 'I'm done. I give up. I've been running and running, and I'm tired. I'm not in control. I want to be, and I've tried to be – my whole life. It doesn't work. I can't do it any more. If you'll have it, take what's left and do with it whatever you want.'

And then, I waited.

I'm not sure what I expected. Anger, maybe. A thunderbolt from above, to finish what I'd begun. The weight of divine silence – or perhaps, nothing at all. In any case, there were no fireworks. No angels or sudden flashes of light – at least, not ones that I could see. But there was something else. Something completely unexpected. I felt a sense of God's overwhelming love. I felt his presence. I felt like he was there. Like he cared for me.

As the wind howled down the chimney, I encountered something that I had never experienced before. A deep, internal quiet. A sense of stillness, like pressing mute on all the background noise.

The day before, I'd been helping my mum pick readings for the funeral. The Bible still lay on the table. I picked it up and opened it at Revelation 1:14. The passage describes Jesus, standing in the throne room of heaven. It sounds fantastical, but these pictures are a way of putting into words a vision that's bigger than speech:

> His head and hair were white like wool, as white as snow, and his eyes were like blazing fire. His feet were like bronze glowing in a furnace, and his voice was like the sound of rushing waters. In his right hand he held seven stars, and out of his mouth came a sharp double-edged sword. His face was like the sun shining in all its brilliance. (Revelation 1:14–16)

As I read, the words sparked and then burst into life. For as long as I could remember, I'd been far too intense. More than anyone could be expected to manage. Too concentrated, too needy, too much.

Yet here was someone else. Someone *more* passionate than me. Here was a vision that caught my breath. Radiant, terrible, beautiful. Irresistible.

A face like the sun. Uncontainable. Blinding. Whose intensity swallowed mine, like candlelight in noonday brilliance.

Eyes that blazed like fire. Who could dare to meet his gaze?

A voice like rushing waters. What words could I add?

Before me stands the living God. Those eyes. That voice. No masks or performances can keep him at bay. In the power of his gaze, I see myself and I want to die. He penetrates every defence, every veneer. He sees me – but he doesn't frown or flinch.

I'm pinned before him. He sees me as I am, and he doesn't walk away. He stares me down, and he doesn't blink.

I am known. Perfectly and entirely. I am *known*.

And so, like John, I fall on my face before him.

Yet he's not done. He picks me up. He lifts my chin and looks me in the eyes. He touches me, like he touched John, and this is what he says: 'Do not be afraid. I am the First and the Last. I am the Living One; I was dead, and behold I am alive for ever and ever! And I hold the keys of death and Hades' (Revelation 1:17–18).

Here at last is a God who's bigger than my drives. A Person, in whose intensity I can rest. Here is the answer to every question:

'Does life matter?'

Yes.

'Have I any value?'

Yes.

'Can I know forgiveness?'

Yes.

'Can I be known and loved?'

Yes, yes, yes. A million times, yes!

Here is a Lord who stoops down. Who stretches out his hand and who whispers, 'Do not be afraid.'

Here is Jesus.

The God who breaks

Shaking, I turned the pages to Revelation 5. I found another picture of the Saviour – one that was just as compelling, yet utterly different. It reads: 'Do not weep! See, the Lion of the tribe of Judah . . . has triumphed' (Revelation 5:5).

My fingers gripped the page as I prepared to meet this lion: a glorious, roaring conqueror. But that's not how the passage continues. Verse 6 says this: 'Then I saw a Lamb, looking as if it had been slain, standing in the centre of the throne.'

It's the same Person. But the Lion is now described as a Lamb.

So who is this Jesus? He's the God who defies our expectations.

He's the Creator of the universe – and he's a bleeding and bow-legged lamb. He's the embodiment of strength and glory – but also of frailty and pain. He's Jesus as Lord, the conquering Lion. And he's Jesus as Lamb, sacrificed and broken.

He's a Monarch, brooking neither rivals nor resistance. He's also a Servant, stooping below the lowest station. He's the Son of God and he's the Son of Man. He understands how it feels to be weak and ashamed and lonely and despised. He's the Lion who dies as a Lamb.

At the centre of the Christian faith stands a very strange symbol. The cross. It represents weakness and torture and shame: the death of a criminal, not a king. It's a picture of the God who comes *to die*. Isn't this slightly . . . well, obscene?

Why choose this death? Why not another? One that's a little safer. More . . . sanitized. Or, even better, tucked away, out of sight. In fact, why die at all? Surely success is about power and glory? Who wants a God who dies in disrepute?

Who wants this God?

Me. I do.

For someone like me, someone broken and crushed by sin and shame, he's not just a good option. He's the only possible Saviour.

Driven and self-willed, I thought that *I* was passionate – but before this great Lion, I'm the one who looks away.

In my self-inflicted misery, I thought *I'd* plumbed the depths, but the slain Lamb goes deeper than I can ever fathom.

A Lamb who meets me in my brokenness. A Lion who vanquishes all my foes. A God who turns his face towards me and says, 'You're mine. I've bought you and that's enough.'

'That's enough.' What does this mean? Enough fighting and striving and hiding and running. Enough starving. Not a question. Not a request. An unalterable fact.

Moments earlier, such words would have filled me with terror. Now, they were accompanied by the thrill of hope. For the first time, I felt that I had an identity. I had a purpose. It wasn't what I'd thought or expected, but that was OK. I wasn't in charge – but I'd met the One who was. The God who could satisfy all of my longings and all of my hungers. Before him, I could hand over control and not be destroyed. *He* was enough, and he wanted me.

The God who gives

I thought that strength meant refusing to serve. But this Jesus confronted me, *not* as a tyrant or heavenly taskmaster, but as a gift. He came *offering himself*. And everything was changed by this truth. On the cross my badness and my goodness were taken away: rendered irrelevant by his sacrifice. He didn't want apologies, resolutions or assurances that I would do better. He wanted *me*. Instead of making me perform, he lifted me clean out of the arena. In return, he asked only one question: Would I *receive* him?

I thought for a moment about what this meant. I'd tried to ring-fence my world with rules and rituals – systems to make life safe. But I'd never understood what it was to receive. I was the girl who always said 'No'.

'No' to people
'No' to relationships
'No' to marriage and health and family and food
'No' to risk and desire and vulnerability and need
'No' to a gospel that I couldn't earn
'No' to a God who was bigger than me – who wanted my heart, not my good intentions

In the past, I'd turned over a thousand new leaves. I'd made a hundred new beginnings, each doomed to failure. These resolutions were all about me – my rules, my strength, my gospel, my way. In the end, I lost all I tried to keep. I got exactly what I asked for: religion without relationship, and law without love. But it left me hungrier than before.

Real repentance

In Romans 2 there's a verse that I've never understood. It says this: 'God's kindness leads you towards repentance' (2:4).

My version of repentance had no room for kindness. Instead, it was about fear, pride and self-will. My version said, 'Pull yourself together. Try harder, do more, make it better. Fix your own mistakes – or face the consequences.'

But real repentance looks very different. It's the product of God's *kindness*, undeserved and poured out without limit. As I stood before the Lord, I expected a fist. He gave me a kiss. What finally floored me was grace. This is what brought me to my knees.

God's *kindness* leads us towards repentance. I couldn't understand it. I couldn't explain it. I couldn't control it. But I couldn't resist it either. Like rain in the desert, it flooded the secret, painful places and left me trembling and changed. My heart thrilled at his voice.

'I love you as you are,' he said, 'but I won't leave you that way. I'm giving you a new start. I'm giving you *a new name*.'

'Shameful.' 'Useless.' 'Weird.' *'Fat.'*

That was my old name.

My new name is something very different. It's something that the Lord is gradually revealing to me. But the Bible gives me some clues.

White stones

Revelation 2:17 tells us that Jesus will give us a 'new name' on the last day. It's a name that's written on a white stone and it's for our eyes only. It's who we really are. And hearing it will be like returning to our native shore after years of exile. Like coming home to everyone you love and finding they're all there. Like rest and wholeness and peace.

This is a wonderful promise, but it's not just for me. The 'new name' is given to *all* of God's people. In Isaiah 62:4 it's the name 'Hephzibah', which is translated: 'My delight is in her.' This is thrilling. It tells us of the Lord's heart leaping with joy when he sees his people. When he looks at me, he is delighted. Not because of my striving, and even in spite of my starving. Not because I hide behind masks or put on a show. The wonder and mystery of the gospel is this: he knows me and yet he loves me. I am completely and irreversibly his.

Meeting the Jesus of the Bible was life-changing. Like Jacob in Genesis 32, I felt as though I'd been fighting and fighting. Finally, he'd won. He'd slain me with his grace. He'd called me to a recovery that was bigger than weight gain: a life, not just an existence. He called me to a relationship with the living God.

In that moment, my world was utterly changed. I understood the gospel: I was forgiven and redeemed. My life had a purpose, and I had a value that was given, not earned. This meant that I could step out of the darkness and uncover my face. I could be broken and messed up. I could admit to my mistakes, my sadness and my guilt. I could find rest in Christ's love. Finally, I could stand and not be shamed.

The verdict

I wasn't who my culture said I was. I wasn't what my family or friends thought either.

I wasn't my job, or my grades. I wasn't my clothes size.

I wasn't my mistakes or my past.

I had an identity, firm and secure.

I was his.

Justice and grace. Majesty and meekness. Strength and love. A Lion and a Lamb.

It's a very different gospel from the one I'd expected – just as he is a very different Lord. But it's so much better than I'd ever dared to dream. And for me, it was a new beginning.

9 Reflections

It's been more than four years since that night in front of the fire. I believe it was a miracle, and I don't say that lightly. But what does a miracle look like? For some, it's an event, a bold leap in the dark. For me, it began a process: a thousand tiny, shuffling steps – not all of them in the right direction.

The first one was this: I started to eat.

I began with 'safe' foods. Vegetables. Fruit, and juice. Then, just as I had cut down on meals, I started to expand them instead. Chicken, cereal, milk: the list went on. Each bite was a breakthrough, but I had constant panic attacks and for months I couldn't sleep. I hated getting bigger – but I felt certain that this was where Jesus was leading me. Despite this, I ricocheted between fury and depression. I wailed and raged and cried – at God, at Glen and at myself.

Some days I went backwards and felt like giving up. I formed new habits: buying only certain brands of food, cleaning (spotless) surfaces, stockpiling groceries. These needed to be challenged, yet there were victories too. An unmade bed. A hot chocolate. Meals out with Glen. A gentle walk along the seafront. Tiptoes towards recovery.

But learning to eat has been just the beginning. Just as diet is only a part of anorexia, so recovery is about more than food. Therefore, getting better is not a simple switch in direction, like changing buses. Instead, it's like turning a massive tanker in the ocean: slow, grinding and arduous. I want to say, 'I'm there: I've done it!' But it's an ongoing process.

Freedom from anorexia is more than looking better or gaining weight. It's about receiving: from God and from others. It's learning to speak out instead of keeping it in. It's resting instead of earning. It's making mistakes. Most of all, recovery is more than choosing not to die. Instead, it's about learning how to live.

I'd like to tell you that today my life is perfect. That getting better is straightforward: painless and quick. Of course that's not true. There are – and have been – many struggles. Here are just a few:

Handling shame

Shame is what drove me to anorexia, but then it kept me there. I starved to escape it, but embodied it instead.

'Shame' is a word you lift out of the vocab box with kid gloves. It's the real deal. Not awkwardness or embarrassment or discomfort. A deep burning in the pit of your stomach. An 'I want to turn myself inside out and climb into the wardrobe and cover myself in coats, and put my hands on my head and then screw my eyes tightly closed and shrink a bit more' kind of feeling.

Unlike more sociable emotions, shame feels personal. It's hard to believe that normal people could catch it. Anger, for example, has a kind of glamour. But shame mopes around corners and grows behind the wallpaper. Shame is never appropriate in polite company. It's a brand, a stamp, a stain. It makes you want to give up and crawl away and hide and apologize until your speech dries up. It's a lowered gaze, a shuffle, an internal folding. It sets you apart, and you can't go back.

Shame has long bony fingers that won't let you go. It clings like a mist and blinds when you least expect it. It's in the stare of others. The neighbour who shook his head every morning as you jogged past. The knowing shop assistants who watched as you filled your basket with lettuce. You pretended not to see them whispering as you left. The pitying glances. The scorn. You could read their thoughts: *What's wrong with her? She's disgusting.*

How do you deal with it? You flee back home, and close the door, tightly. But you can't outrun yourself. Years later, you wonder: Where does that crazy girl go? Is she still there, wandering empty-handed through the aisles? Poised, but infinitely patient. Watching. Waiting.

Here's what I want to do to her. I'd like to lock her in a box. I'd like to toss her in the ocean and delete her name from my address list and pepper her full of bullets and then run her over – just to make sure. But I can't. 'She' is me. And while her behaviour has changed, she won't be silenced.

So what do I tell her? *'Try harder'*?

What do I do with my disgrace?

Part of resisting shame is recognizing that I want it too. It serves a purpose. It tells me I'm too disgusting to engage with God or the world. And that's attractive. If I withdraw into self-hatred, I can kill my desires and suppress my regrets. Shame helps me close down the hope I dare not feel – hope that I might be accepted and loved after all. It's a neat way of punishing myself for the years I've wasted, the choices I've made and the damage I can't reverse.

Shame is the shape of an eating disorder. It 'works' like this: I know I'm not OK, but *I'll* say why and *I'll* prescribe my own cure. I'll identify what's wrong in me, and I will fix it.

The way of Jesus is very different. *He* – not my 'fat', my 'former life' or even me – is the sacrifice for my sins. *He* is the scapegoat and *he* deals with the mess. Jesus takes my shame and offers me himself.

Being real

The grace of Jesus gives me the strength to be weak. He gives me permission to speak as someone who *struggles*, not someone who pretends. Against my natural instincts, I've started being honest about who I am. This happened with close friends first. Then at church. I've told my story at seminars and conferences. And I write every day, especially on my blog. As someone who's used to hiding in the dark, it's been quite a turnaround. So why do it? Why fix my name to something so ugly?

There are many reasons. I want to make sense of the world. To encourage and be encouraged. To testify to Christ's love and power. To remind myself of where I've come from, so that, by his grace, I never go back. And finally, to unmask the impostor of shame.

I hate anorexia, and I don't want to be associated with it. But more than this, I hate its secrecy and its lies. As I write and speak about it, I'm fighting it as best I can. I'm trying to expose it, as it tried to expose me.

My temptation is to cover up and act strong. But more and more, I'm seeing that real power lies in vulnerability and openness. I've met others who struggle – through my website and at conferences. As we speak with honesty about our darkest battles, *that's* when the shame begins to recede.

Jesus says to Paul, 'My grace is sufficient for you, for my power is made perfect in weakness.' I long to respond as Paul does, with these words: 'Therefore I will boast all the more gladly about my weaknesses, so that Christ's power may rest on me' (2 Corinthians 12:9).

Handling the fallout

I am very weak – not just in spirit, but in body too. As I starved my body, I felt invincible – but anorexia has left me with some lasting scars. Sadly, I'm not alone. The longer the disorder lasts, the more it costs. For some, these consequences can be reversed with weight gain. But not for all.

I've been a healthy weight for several years now, but it's unlikely that I'll return to the person I was. I've got limited strength, and am less mobile than many grannies. My gums are receding and my immunity is poor. I used to love running, but even short walks can be too much. I've got osteopenia (the beginning of osteoporosis), and I tire very quickly.

My brain limps too. Like an old computer, if I open too many programmes (or try to do too much), it freezes and shuts down. Sometimes I'll get 'stuck' trying to do basic tasks or make simple decisions. My short-term memory is patchy, and I find it hard to concentrate, even on the books I used to love.

Then there's my digestive system.

When I started eating again, it was hard to process certain foods and I felt bloated and nauseous. I figured that my body would eventually adjust. Unfortunately, that hasn't been the case.

After years of inactivity, my bowels don't coordinate the way they should. Put baldly, this means that I can't go to the toilet without mechanical help. I'd love to spare you the details – but this is the real face of an eating disorder. When I started to eat, my system backed up and I became very sick. The doctors were worried that my intestines would burst, and I was hospitalized on a number of occasions.

Since then, we've considered all sorts of options, from radical surgery to a permanent colostomy bag. None have held much appeal! Working with specialists, we've found strategies for mechanically moving things along, but they can leave me feeling drained and nauseous. It's also time-consuming and embarrassing. My consultant has treated victims of torture, and said that my insides have failed in just the same way as theirs. Of course, there's one big difference. They were victims; I did this to myself.

A related struggle has been with massive bloating. Some fluid retention is normal as your body gets used to processing food – but it usually passes. We assumed that my bowels would get better, but instead they got worse. This means that, when my stomach distends, I look like

I'm pregnant. And not just a little pregnant either – I've had to wear maternity trousers, and even walking can be difficult. I'm not being oversensitive: I've been given cards of congratulation, and my GP has asked me to take multiple pregnancy tests, 'just to make sure'. Sometimes people volunteer their bus seats, but that's been the only plus. I've got stretch marks – but no baby.

This hurts.

I've longed to be a mother for as long as I can remember. But, despite regaining weight, it might not ever be possible. Sometimes when I think about it, I'm OK. Sometimes I'm really not: I see a small child and I'm winded, like being punched in the stomach.

It raises big and painful questions, about who I am and where I place my hope. Questions like these:

How does a workaholic react when the plug is pulled? Having defined myself through performance, how do I cope when simply getting out of a chair is exhausting? How do I make sense of the past? Am I allowed to feel grief, or only guilt?

Without an eating disorder, a job, a family or a healthy body, is there anyone left? If so, who is she? Does she have a future? Or like Peter Pan, is she locked forever in her past?

Handling my feelings

One theory behind eating disorders is that sufferers are afraid of growing up. To me, this makes sense. I felt like a child, and so I became one. My periods stopped. My curves disappeared. I pressed pause on my body and succeeded in freezing time.

Over the years, I drifted into anorexia and then sank, far beneath the water, where I felt warm and safe. I stopped trying to swim – until someone tugged at the lifeline and pulled me, gasping and crying through the surface. When I began to eat, it was as though the clock was starting again. Like gulping lungfuls of cold air, there were people and noise and shouting, and everything was too sharp and too fast. I felt as though I was an infant, learning to speak and eat and feel, as if for the first time. I didn't want to go back in the water – but I'd forgotten how to walk.

Even when your body matures, it can take time for your affections to catch up. That's because anorexia is bigger than biology: there's an emotional regression too. Without your eating disorder, you have to re-enter the world, all over again. You rediscover a place outside the womb you've created, and people beyond yourself.

It's hard to explain: you're thirty-something, but you're also thirteen. You never learned how to manage your feelings, and now they're All Here and Shouting at each other, like uncles at a wedding. You're happy and sad and lonely and shy and hopeful and despairing, and a million other things that won't be covered by the adjective 'fat'.

You're used to watching life from a distance, with the sound on mute. But now, those emotions are back – as raw and as urgent as ever.

Some of them are good. Some are bad. All of them are frightening.

Handling hungers

First, your appetites. It's a real shock: giving your body something that it actually wants. Caring for and feeding it, after years of abuse. Learning to eat. A mouthful of terror, rising in your throat. But with it, relief. And something else. Pleasure.

The taste – oh, the taste of food! The wonder of biting into something and enjoying it. An apple. A glass of milk. Raisin bread, smeared with butter and strawberry jam. The feel of it in your mouth. Like flowers bursting into bloom.

When you start to feed, it's like opening the floodgates on years of hunger. You're gripped by the desire to stuff yourself and never stop.

Here's the question: How do people eat? It's basic, but so difficult. The chewing and swallowing and leaving it there in your tummy. You're bewildered and terrified by what it might do. How do you recognize when you're hungry and when you're full? What constitutes a 'normal' portion of food?

After so long on lettuce, the options are overwhelming. 'Bad' foods are now 'good'. Your brain says 'No', while your body shrieks, 'Yes. YES!' Up to 60% of recovering anorexics struggle with binge-eating or bulimia: it's hard to find a balance when you've denied yourself for so long.

Managing my appetite continues to be a challenge, though it has become easier. To begin with, I felt stuffed after just a few bites. Later, I couldn't stop. I still confuse my physical and emotional hungers – especially when I'm anxious or stressed. I'm still tempted to see food as the answer to my problems – but in reverse. Where I used to starve myself to feel in control, occasionally I'm tempted to binge-eat instead. This has a physical dimension – carbohydrates, for example, have a soothing effect. There's something else too: that lingering desire to prove I'm better and to fix things by 'finishing my plate'.

When I was at uni, we had an elevated table, reserved for special guests. Sometimes when I eat with others, I'm reminded of that table. On bad days, I'm still tempted to see food as a performance, a barometer of worth. Of course, this is in my head. But unless I fight it, it'll determine my behaviour too. It'll shame me all over again.

It's one thing to spot faulty thinking. It's another to break the habits of a lifetime. To start with, calories felt dirty and unfamiliar, like intruders, triggering a million internal alarms. I was seized by panic after eating, and those first meals sat in my stomach like a sack of cement. My body was changing. Expanding. Some of this was good. My hair grew back. I had more energy and felt less cold. I was able to concentrate – on films, conversations and people. But it was tough as well. For a long time, I couldn't look in the mirror. In the shower, I'd still scrub at my flesh. Old clothes were too small – but new ones too big. Physically, I was more alert. Mentally, I felt shattered. I was swollen with questions as well as with food.

How do you live as a physical person? And what does it mean to take care of your body?

What's fluid retention and what is weight gain? Why do I feel so sick? How do I know when I'm full? What does an 'average' meal look like? Will my periods return?

Why am I so angry and depressed? Will I ever feel normal again?

In my darker moments, I thought about killing myself.

'Lord!' I cried. 'Help me. Help me.'

Handling the middle ground

I longed to take a pill and wake up 'better'. But it doesn't work like that. There's no schedule for recovery: no fast-forward, and no rewind. In the relentless pursuit of thinness, there was no time to think. Without this, time became a sentence to be served.

My body, processing an alien sustenance, felt sluggish and heavy. My brain – too shredded to settle – lurched haphazardly from one scheme to another. I was manic – and lethargic. I wanted to run the planet – but I couldn't get out of bed. Sometimes I tried to read, but the sentences ran into each other. I'd switch on the TV, but all I could see were shows about cookery and slimming. When I went out, there were people and noise and lights, and they crashed over me and knocked me off my feet. Nothing made sense, and I longed for the old slaveries, for safety and routines to buttress the panic.

Over time, however, God's promises began to sink in. I did jigsaws, listened to music and made lists of the things I used to enjoy. This helped – but I was plagued by internal voices, and they all said different things. Which ones should I trust?

Mentally and emotionally, I was exhausted. Physically, I could do a little more. In itself, this was dangerous: I'd always pushed beyond the bounds of possibility and 'a little more' never felt like enough. But to break the cycle of burnout, I had to change. So I picked up the threads of old friendships and initiated new ones. I plugged in my computer and started answering the phone. I stopped hiding – my weight, my diet, my movements. This took time: I'd grown used to lying, and it was a hard habit to break. But it was progress, nonetheless. Loved ones began to exhale. 'She's getting better. Finally, finally.' They were right. But getting better made me *feel* much worse.

I started to look normal again. Other people didn't stare so much. But they were still watching. Those quick up-and-down assessments. The unspoken questions: *Is she losing weight? How long will it last?* Family and friends, poised like hawks. Enough elephants in the room to start a circus.

There's no protocol for an eating disorder. People aren't sure what to say, and neither are you. Well meaning, they fumble towards speech. 'Your cheeks are filling out. You look . . . healthier.'

Of course they mean 'fatter', but you smile and nod. 'Yes,' you say. 'I'm fine.'

But you're not. You want to tell them, 'I need *more* support now and not less.' But the words stick in your throat.

You're scared and angry and sad. You want to let people in, but you don't know how. With one hand, you're pushing them away; with another, you're pulling them in. You're caught between loneliness and fear: frightened of what they'll see, but also of being alone.

Does recovery get easier? Yes – but the timetable's not fixed. Nor is the shape. There are, however, many helps as well as struggles. Here are a few of mine:

'Ordinary' people

It's hard hearing from the experts that your problems are too big. It's easy to give up hope. Friends and family worried that they were too inexperienced to help. But their support was crucial. More than we needed 'answers', we needed people to love us and to stand with us in our mess. We needed 'ordinary' people, not just professionals. What do they look like?

My beautiful husband. Patient, wise, funny, strong. I could fill a million books with the ways he's carried me. Just thinking about him swells my heart.

Our families, loyal and loving.

Our church, who wooed us back into relationship.

Old friends from school and university who remind us of who we are.

New friends, who embrace us, in all our mess. Strangers who prayed for us and let us stay at their homes. A godly vicar and his wife. Gracious women who modelled to me strong, gentle femininity – and kept asking me out for coffee, even when I (repeatedly) cancelled. Saints (and sinners) who prayed for us – and still do. A supportive bishop. Belgian friends, who became partners in crime. Neighbours who quietly weeded, cat-sat and served us in hundreds of ways.

These people saved our lives. But medical help was a necessary part of recovery too. I was used to seeing doctors as enemies, convinced that they'd lock me up and throw away the key. Such fears had to be faced. With Glen's help, I registered with a doctor, had a full check-up, explained my history and asked for support. I had blood tests, bone scans, weigh-ins and fertility tests. I went to a local group for those recovering from eating disorders. I read books on recovery, and tried to learn from those who'd walked the same paths. Most of all, I prayed, prayed and prayed again. And when I couldn't pray, other people did it for me.

Community

Just as anorexia impacts on your relationships, so recovery will involve those around you too. They're allies who will fight for you when you're too weak to fight for yourself. They'll reveal things that you can't see alone. They'll minister to you as individuals, and as a couple too.

Three years ago, Glen and I met just such a group. We went to a conference run by Larry Crabb, and felt nervous and unsure of what to expect. What we found was extraordinary: a group of very different people, speaking with astonishing honesty about their struggles. It was light that illuminated our marriage: painful, but liberating too. We came to see disordered dynamics within our relationship that pulled us both down. The interaction of sufferer and carer is sometimes overlooked in recovery, but it's absolutely vital.

In his book, *Telling Secrets*, Frederick Buechner describes how he learned to handle his daughter's anorexia:

> The only way I knew to be a father was to take care of
> her, as my father had been unable to take care of me,
> to move heaven and earth if necessary to make her well,
> and of course I couldn't do that. I didn't have either the
> wisdom or the power to make her well. None of us has
> the power to change other human beings like that,
> and it would be a terrible power if we did, the power
> to violate the humanity of others even for their own
> good . . .

Buechner came to see that, much as he longed to, he could not 'fix' his daughter. Indeed, it would not be right for *either* of them if he did.

If your daughter is struggling for life in a raging torrent, you do not save her by jumping into the torrent with her, which leads only to your both drowning together. Instead you keep your feet on the dry bank – you maintain as best you can your own inner peace, the best and strongest of who you are – and from that solid ground reach out a rescuing hand . . . A bleeding heart is of no help to anybody if it bleeds to death.[4]

As others opened up to us, Glen and I saw the truth about ourselves. We'd allowed anorexia to define our marriage: 'us' as well as me. I had taken on the role of sufferer, but Glen too had invested in a counterfeit identity – as my rescuer. By casting himself as a burden-bearing ox, he needed a burden to bear. But instead of rescuing me, he was crushed instead.

The grace that changes

For Glen and I to move forward, we needed to make a fresh start. One afternoon we sat down and wrote each other a letter. In these letters, we listed all the things we'd done (or not done) which had harmed the other one. We read them aloud and asked each other for forgiveness. Then we burned them and prayed, asking God to help us move forward.

Confessing our sins in the presence of love – *this* is what changes us. Not our performance, not our masks, not our gifts. Whatever the issue – addiction, eating disorders, abuse, hurt, anger, shame – it's grace that transforms.

A final feast

I was reminded of this yesterday, as I watched two friends getting married. I'd been running late on this book, and Glen had sermons to write, so we weren't planning to linger. After the service, we ducked into the reception. As we congratulated the happy couple, they asked us to stay – but I'd already eaten, and the three-course menu was not friendly to my digestive problems.

My inner perfectionist awoke, tugging me back to my deadline and the security of home. But, as we looked around at the friends gathered there, we smiled and took off our coats. Old Emma would have run a mile. The new Emma prayed, and left her book preparation and digestive tract in the Lord's hands.

As we ate together and toasted the happy couple, I was overwhelmed by gratitude at where the Lord had brought us to. It was a little taste of the final banquet where Christ himself will be head of the table. A feast I can't wait to attend – and to share with you.

I've spent most of my life trying to be someone I'm not. Someone I could be proud of – who looks and acts 'right'. Someone with answers, achievements and a system for managing life. Someone 'in control'. Does this 'someone' even exist? No! And she's not meant to, either.

Jesus has shown me someone more precious than the perfect me. Finally, he has given me the name and the identity I've always longed for.

> Everyone who wins the victory will be made into a pillar in the temple of my God, and they will stay there for ever. I will write on each of them the name of my God and the name of his city. It is the new Jerusalem that my God will

send down from heaven. I will also write on them my own new name.

Listen! I am standing and knocking at your door. If you hear my voice and open the door, I will come in and we will eat together.
(Revelation 3:12, 20 CEV)

Notes

1. Louis MacNeice, 'Snow', *Selected Poems* (Faber and Faber, 2007).
2. See Marilyn Duker and Roger Slade, *Anorexia Nervosa and Bulimia: How to Help*, 2nd edn (Open University Press, 2002).
3. Stevie Smith, 'Not Waving but Drowning', *The Collected Poems of Stevie Smith* (Penguin, 1972).
4. Frederick Buechner, *Telling Secrets* (Harper San Francisco, 1991), pp. 26–27.

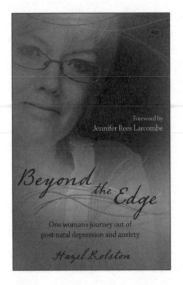

Beyond the Edge

*One woman's journey
out of post-natal
depression and anxiety*
Hazel Rolston

ISBN: 9781844742165
160 pages, paperback

'Broken, desperate and humiliated, I entered the house.
When I saw Steve and Katherine, my heart felt like it was
going to explode in agony. They did not deserve this madness
in their lives ...'

Cut off by a dense fog of post-natal depression and anxiety,
Hazel Rolston felt pushed beyond the edge. But when the
grim voice of Despair offered her the path of suicide, she
knew instinctively that this was not God's way for her.

Hazel doesn't offer us a formula for instant escape. But she
does remind us that God is there, even if our feelings say
the opposite. No matter how bad things feel, God is faithful
to his wounded, broken people beyond the edge.

'As Hazel lays bear her heart, we discover, not slogans or
rhetoric, but authentic hope. This gritty, immensely readable
book is more than a tonic. It's a lifesaver.' Jeff Lucas

'Read this book and be changed to reach out with Jesus'
compassion.' Alie Stibbe

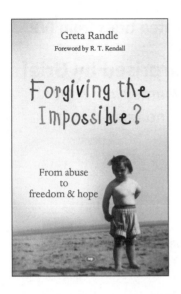

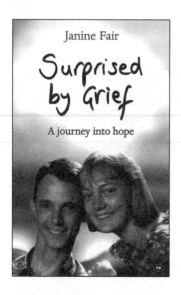

related titles from IVP

Surprised by Grief
A journey into hope
Janine Fair

ISBN: 9781844744725
144 pages, paperback

'Losing a partner at a young age is a devastating experience. I know. I've been there.'

Janine shares the agonizing emotions, and the inner journey God took her on, after her biggest nightmare became reality literally overnight. She looks at the traps and pitfalls to which she was particularly prone, along with the overwhelming sense of loneliness she felt. And she shares the long and gruelling path towards recovering her sense of self and forging a new identity.

'God led me to set new priorities for myself,' she says, *'as I sought to move into the future with him, and enabled me to deal with the baggage of negative beliefs.'*

Finally, Janine places her grief in the context of a transition in order to understand her 'voyage of hope', ending with gratitude to God for all she has received from his hands.

Available from your local Christian bookshop or **www.thinkivp.com**

discover more great Christian books
at www.ivpbooks.com

Full details of all the books from Inter-Varsity Press – including
reader reviews, author information, videos and free downloads –
are available on our website at **www.ivpbooks.com**.

IVP publishes a wide range of books on various subjects including:

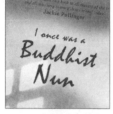

Biography

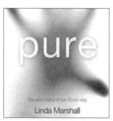

Christian Living

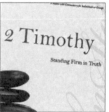

Bible Studies

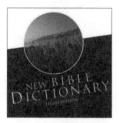

Reference

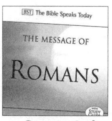

Commentaries

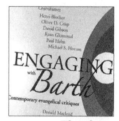

Theology

On the website you can also sign up for regular email newsletters,
tell others what you think about books you have read by posting
reviews, and locate your nearest Christian bookshop using the
Find a Store feature.

IVP publishes Christian books that are **true to the Bible**
and that **communicate the gospel, develop discipleship**
and **strengthen the church** for its mission in the world.